LESSER KNOWN FORMS
OF
PERFORMING ARTS IN INDIA

LESSER KNOWN FORMS
OF
PERFORMING ARTS IN INDIA

compiled and edited
by
DURGADAS MUKHOPADHYAY

STERLING PUBLISHERS PVT LTD
AB/9 Safdarjang Enclave, New Delhi-110016

Distributed in the USA by
International Publications Service, Inc.,
114 East 32nd Street, New York; N.Y. 10016

ISBN 0 8426 1004 9

Lesser Known Forms of Performing Arts in India
ⓒ 1978, Durgadas Mukhopadhyay
Copyright for individual articles with their respective authors.
Published by S.K. Ghai, Managing Director, Sterling Publishers (P) Ltd.,
AB/9, Safdarjang Enclave, New Delhi-110016 and printed at Sterling
Printers, L-11, Green Park Extn., New Delhi-110016
35/4/1978

*to the expert exponents
of traditional performances
languishing in remote villages of India*

PREFACE

How little do we know of our tradition! How little do we care! Some only speak of it, others frown. The need is to imbibe the essentials of our tradition for a smooth cultural growth able to sustain shocks and chaos in the future.

The urge to express, to communicate, to share something beautiful gave birth to performing arts. The living progressive impulse to the timeless universal gets shape in creative designs. Tradition plays an important role in creative artistic processes, particularly in the field of performing art.

This book is the first in a series of volumes on traditional performances in India. An attempt is made to document and analyse the hitherto unexplored mosaic of the potent lesser-known forms of performing arts in India. The aim is to document various lesser-known forms of classical, folk and tribal dance, theatre, music and painting traditions which are potent, aesthetically invigorating, in different states of India. The articles are research-oriented serious studies taking into account the various facets of performing arts—historical, sociological, anthropological or ritual, economic and administrative, aesthetic and technical aspects in a pre-designed compact format. Various gurus and exponents were consulted, interviewed and materials were collected from fieldwork in different regions to enrich the contents in a spirit of cooperative venture.

The guiding principle has been to trace the history or origin of a particular form, its growth and transformation. The socio-economic factors behind its decay are analysed. The ritual, anthropological and regional aspects are considered in detail in a comparative framework. A representative performance popular in the region is elaborately described from beginning to the end of the programme—the story-line, the costume, make-up, masks, instruments, dance movements, songs in original and translation, *tala*, *laya*, stagecrafts, etc. alongwith photographs of the performances or the overview of the stage. Finally, the relevance, necessity, possibility of restoration, revival, adaptation and assimilation is considered in detail.

Recent attempts at revival and institutional assistance and professional interest is outlined. We strongly believe that a potent tradition would survive the onslaught of neon lights, fashion and commercialisation.

We have included three articles on Jatra, Tamasha and Powada—rather well known and popular forms—to highlight the extent of thematic, technical and conceptual vulgarisation in the name of modernisation and the harm it has done to the structural unity and aesthetic appeal of traditional performances.

The folk-theatre is changing its structure continuously over centuries, modifying itself to the needs of changing situations making it functionally relevant to the society. At present the urban art-forms with the limitations and dead-end future is exploring new grounds in folk-tradition. The powerful and viable forms must be restored to their former glory and meaningfulness keeping in mind that they must be functional in the future. A little more awareness, sympathy and patronage from discerning connoisseurs would be sufficient. These forms had been an integral part of the process of living of the masses. The essentially human element is being lost in the age of machines imposing limitations on the spontaneity and freedom of design and the imagination of the creative artist.

As Ananda K. Coomaraswamy puts it : "The first expression of national idealism is then a rehabilitation of the past." In order to "defend the Prolific against the Devourer" one must go through "a process of creative introspection preparatory to activity." This process does not imply a revival of the past and return to it, since "we must make our home in the future." "Still the future has to be built on our love for the past and on our passionate conviction about its value."

We have a lot to learn from the traditional forms of performing arts and much to share with the fellow thinkers from different regions of India. Let there be an interchange of ideas among the connoisseurs in different parts of India. The book hopes to serve as a reference manual for academicians, performers, critics and connoisseurs with its in-depth interdisciplinary analysis.

Durgadas Mukhopadhyay

CONTENTS

ACKNOWLEDGEMENTS

I would like to thank my friends Keshav Malik, Mala Marwah, Mayadhar Rout, Jaipal Singh for assistance received at various stages of preparing this volume. I am grateful to the editor of *Sangeet Natak* for permission to include four articles which appeared earlier in their journal—"Mask Dances of Bengal ": Dr Asutosh Bhattacharya, "Veethi Bhagavatam" : Dr V. Raghavan, "Yakshagana Bayalata" : K.S. Upadhyaya, "Gotipua Dancers of Orissa ": Sunil Kothari. Grateful acknowledgement is due to the editor of *Quarterly Journal of National Centre for Performing Arts* for permission to include the article on "Powada" : Dr Ashok Ranade, published earlier in their journal. Pria Karunakar had helped in the whole project with sympathy, understanding and heart-felt cooperation.

D.M.

ABOUT THE CONTRIBUTORS

D. Appukuttan Nair : A reputed connoisseur of the traditional visual arts of Kerala. Founder of **Margi**—art society devoted to traditional art-forms.

Dr G. Sankara Pillai : is Professor of Malayalam and President of Kerala Sangeet Natak Akademi. Written books on performing arts in Kerala.

Kavalam Narayana Panicker : Award-winning playwright. Former Secretary of the Kerala Sangeet Natak Akademi.

Dr V.S. Sharma : Professor of Malayalam in Kerala University. Did his doctoral dissertation on "Thullal Art Form in Kerala."

K.C. Sharma : is the special representative of Haryana Government in Delhi.

Sharbari Mukherjee : Vocalist, Writer. Works with N.C.E.R.T.

Dr Asutosh Bhattacharya : Director, Folk Art Research Centre, Calcutta.

Dr V. Raghavan : Well-known scholar of classical dance and theatre forms.

Ratnadhar Jha : Journalist working with *Hindustan Times.* Published books and articles on Mithila Painting and Literature.

Dr Om Prakash Joshi : Lecturer, Rajasthan University. Currently engaged in Post-Doctoral Research in Department of Sociology, Delhi University.

Dhyaneshwar Nadkarni : Well-known journalist from Bombay.

Dr Ashok Ranade : Head of the Department of Music and Fine Arts, Bombay University.

Kalamandalam Kalyanikutty Amma : Noted exponent of Mohiniattam.

K.S. Upadhyaya : Well-known journalist from Karnataka.

Durgadas Mukhopadhyay : Poet, Playwright, Critic. Lecturer, Delhi University. Currently working on 'Tribal Culture in India'.

Dr Krishna Bisht : Vocalist. Lecturer, Department of Music, Delhi University.

Dhiren Pattanaik : Secretary, Orissa State Sangeet Natak Akademi. Written books and articles on Odissi and folk dances of Orissa.

Sadhashiva Ratha Sharma : Noted authority on traditional performing arts in Orissa.

A. Chowdhury : Free-lance Journalist.

Ashok Chakradhar : Lecturer in Hindi, Jamia Millia. Produced and directed a number of Nautanki plays.

Sunil Kothari : Journalist from Bombay.

Jiwan Pani : Works with the Sangeet Natak Akademi, New Delhi. Written articles on folk art forms of Eastern India.

1

KOODIYATTOM

D. Appukkuttan Nair

Koodiyattom, the unique temple art of Kerala, is probably the only surviving form of the traditional presentation of Sanskrit drama. The performance is confined to the temple theatres known as Koothambalams, the performing artistes belong to specific temple dependent communities known as Chakkiars and Nambiars. The Chakkiars are the actors and the Nangiars of the Nambiar community undertake female roles to the accompaniment of the Mizhavus (pot-like drums covered with animal hide) and Edakka (a small drum played with a stick), Kurumkuzhal (a small wind instrument similar to a Shehnai) and Kuzhithalam (a small pair of cymbals).

The Sanskrit plays—usually presented on the stage, belong mainly to those of the Trivandrum Sanskrit series, namely, those of Bhasa, Kulasekhara Varman, Sree Harshan, Mahendra-vikrama Pallavan and Bodhayanan, apart from *Ascharya Choodamani* by the Kerala dramatist Shakti Bhadran.

The Koodiyattom as it is presented today was choreographed some ten centuries ago by King Kulasekhara Varman with the assistance of his friend Tholan. The form of presentation is highly stylised in *Aharya Abhinaya* (make-up, costume and scenic spectacle), *Angika Abhinaya* (gesture) and *Vachika Abhinaya* (oral rendering). There is no attempt at realism. In fact, the attempt is to represent Puranic characters in a super-human form, in an epic setting—nor can we claim a close adherence to the canons laid down in Natya Sastra in the presentation of this dramatic art form.

In Angika Abhinaya, in which Hastha Mudras are liberally used in descriptions, conversations, and dissertations, the Lakshanas codified in Natya Sastra or the various other texts in Hindu dramaturgy are not faithfully followed. The Hastha Mudras are taken from *Hastha Lakshana Deepika* which draws from the Tŗantric mudras prevalent in Kerala. The other movements of the body, belonging to the Angika Abhinaya particularly the Charis, Gatis and the movements of the various Angas and Upangas of the body also do not closely follow the canons prescribed by the Natya Sastra.

In Aharya Abhinaya the make up and costumes do not copy the external features of the characters either in facial make up, head gear, clothing or ornament. The make up is symbolic of the nature of the character presented on the stage. At the same time, there is no typifying of characters as in Kathakali. While in Kathakali, Bali and Sugreeva wear the same costume, in Koodiyattom, their costumes are different. Bali, as the more kind and powerful of the two, possessing noble traits of character with certain aspects of amorous expression towards Tara, has make-up which brings out those characteristics.

In Vachika Abhinaya, the text of the Sanskrit drama is rendered by the actor with intonations reminding us of the Yajur-Vedic chantings of the Nambudiri Brahmins of Kerala. There is no attempt at making the speeches naturalistic. Even ragas (*swaras* as they are called in Koodiyattom) do not have the solfa symbols of music. The prose renderings also abound in certain intonations, which make for greater stylisation.

Koodiyattom plays are not presented in full. Presentation is so elaborate and there are such lengthy excursions into various fields that it makes presentation time-consuming. Hence nowadays these plays are presented only in part—each part being known by a different name. Thus, Swapnavasavadatta is presented as six different performances, each performance confining itself to one *Anka* (One Act). These Ankas (Acts) are also known by different names. Thus in Swapnavasavadatta the Ankas are called Brahmacharyankam, Pandattankam, Shebhalikankam, Swapnankam, Chithrabhalakankam etc. In Prathigna Nataka, there is one Anka called Manthrankam which takes 41 days to perform. This is an oral exposition by

Vidooshaka of all things under the Sun. Similarly, the Anguliyankam of *Ascharya Choodamani* lasting for twelve full days tells the full story of Ramayana including Vanarolpathi by Shri Hanuman, by hand gestures alone.

Since one Anka (Act) of the drama alone is performed at one time, there is a prelude to this performance called *Nirvahana* during which one of the characters sums up the story presented in the earlier Acts of the drama and possibly the earlier stories. This 'Nirvahana' takes very many days and if this 'Nirvahana' is 'rendered' by the Vidooshaka, it is an oral exposition. Other characters use hand gestures for this purpose.

The performance can be classified into two parts on the basis of the relative importance of the Vidooshaka, the comic character. Thus, performances like the first Act of Subhadradhananjayam, the first Act of Stapathisamvaranam etc., are Vidooshaka dominant where there is greater emphasis on Vachika Abhinaya (oral rendering). The Vidooshaka talks in Malayalam. He interprets the Sanskrit *slokas* recited by the characters in Malayalam and recites parodies of these slokas and expounds the various laws of nature in a very humorous manner.

The most important characteristic of Koodiyattom is its elaborate interpretation of the Sanskrit *slokas* or stanzas through hand gestures by the various characters and by oral expositions of the Vidooshaka. The slokas are enacted in such a way that the inner multiple meanings of the various slokas are explained to the audience. Even incidents, anecdotes and philosophy which have only an indirect and very remote bearing on the meaning of the slokas can be indicated by the actors. In Abhishekanataka in the Thorana Yudha Ankom there is a sloka in which Ravana speculates that the reason for a monkey devastating the palace in Lanka is due to the disrespect he showed to Nandikeswara. Nandikeswara had cursed him, saying that he would be ruined by a monkey. In enacting this sloka the actor describes in detail Ravana's war with the Devas and the Asuras; he details the preparations for the war, the triumphant journey thereafter, a description of Lanka, his expedition to win over Vaishravana and the blocking of Pushpaka Vimana by Mount Kailas, the vivid features of Mount

Kailas, the quarrel between Parvathi and Siva and so on. The Angika Abhinaya of this sloka takes 3 to 4 hours to perform.

Such elaborate and lengthy Abhinaya of the Sanskrit slokas may seem tedious to an indifferent audience. For their entertainment, there are the humorous oral expositions spiced with some vulgarity by the Vidooshaka. The Vidooshaka also expounds the famous Purushartha or the four ultimate attainments in human life. This is a satire on the follies and foibles of human life by which he recounts the exploits of a group of adventurous high caste Hindus to attain the four aims, namely, Rajaseva (waiting upon the King with flattery, gossip, etc.), Asanam (greedy enjoyment of an enormous feast), Vinodam (sexual enjoyment with a prostitute) and Vanchanam (betrayal of the prostitute whom he has enjoyed). These four Purusharthas are interpreted in place of Dharma, Artha, Kama and Moksha. This oral exposition usually takes more than four days, during which there will be much pointed satire at the way of living of highbrow society, involving the audience.

All told, Koodiyattom is unique in its presentation of classical Sanskrit drama through the vitality of the folk medium.

2

THOTTAM

G. Sankara Pillai

Kerala's folk-ritual heritage is as varied and rich as its landscape. Though many of the folk forms have either deteriorated or drifted into oblivion, the rituals and various visual forms associated with them are still reverenced by the rural community. And among these rituals the most important are the ceremonies connected with the 'Mother Goddess worship'. Historians and sociologists have much to say about the apparent predominance of the 'mother cult' in Kerala. The opinion of certain scholars that 'mother worship' came to South India as a result of the Aryan invasion has been effectively disproved by the later writers on the subject. Some of them like Gilbert Slater (in *The Dravidian Element in Indian Culture*) have gone to the other extreme of establishing that Indian culture itself is essentially Dravidian in nature. The sweep of Aryanisation through the indigenous Kerala culture is itself an interesting phenomenon. It has made its owns mark on our customs, rituals, art, way of life and literature. It was not a conquest, the invaders and the invaded coming into direct clash with each other, as happened elsewhere, but a silent, intellectual conquest by which a mutual synthesis was attempted, knowingly or unknowingly. However one result of this is that many indigenous institutions, systems and usages lost their identity, partially or completely, as a result of these attempts. Yet comparatively less harm is done in the realm of religion, evidently because of the element of the supernatural. Aryan culture when it came in contact with the indigenous concept of the Mother Goddess discovered a new Deity. There are many famous 'Devi' temples in the State, but, the establishment of such temples did not in the least destroy the age-old practices of the villager's worship of his favourite Mother Goddess. He called her 'Kali'. Kali is different from 'Durga' or 'Karthyayani'. She is fierce—the incarnation of the villager's concept of the avenger of all evils. If displeased she will inflict corporal punishment on evildoers, most often to the whole village. She will bring small pox; she will destroy her victims as thoroughly as she dealt with 'Darika'. (Kali's incarnation, according to the myth met him at a duel. She tore him, literally to pieces. The *pattu* (song) which describes this in great detail narrates how she tore out his liver and cut it into little pieces for her retinue to swallow; how she did not spare even the small bone in his body !) This concept of the deity has also another equally important phase. If she is pleased, she may be extremely generous; equally powerful in bestowing fertility, good crops, and a prosperous life. The villager is eager to placate her, his presiding deity. At harvest he invokes her to come and be in the village midst. He is ready to offer her his best. He considers her his mother—the Mother of mothers. The Kali concept has sprung really from the villager's reverence to the mother—the propagator of the family, and to mother-earth—his only reliable basis of existence. J.M. Campbell and Herbert Spencer, among others have tried to establish that such ancient practices of worship may have sprung from the worship of the dead—in other words ancestor worship. K.R. Pisharati's 'Cult and Cult acts of Kerala' (*Indian Historical Quarterly*) has divided the worship motifs into (1) the worship of heroes (2) the worship of invisible powers both noble and ignoble (3) the worship of the dead.

Even now in Kerala, many ancient families practise ancestral worship. If we scrutinise the rituals followed in 'Kali' worship it will be evident that they are in fact extensions of the ancestor rituals.

'Thottam' is the ritual connected with indigenous worship of Kali in Kerala. The essence of Thottam means 'restoration to life'. It is derived from 'Thottuka'—to 'invoke' or 'to reincarnate'. Thottam is a ritual which reincarnates the Goddess Kali in a specific place made auspicious for the occasion. The mode of this ritual varies from place to place.   The songs, literature, and ceremonies differ. In the southern most district of Kerala a small hut of green coconut leaves is built amidst the fields, after harvest.   A 'Peedha' will be placed inside covered with a deep red cloth called 'Pattu'.   On it a sword will be placed.   A ballad in praise of the deity depicts in detail her valiant fight with 'Darika' and will be sung by a group either for 7, 14, or 21 days.   This song is called "Thottam Pattu" and the singers are in most cases members of an advanced community—the matriarchal Nairs. There is no script and it is seriously believed that it is extremely dangerous to allow the Thottam Pattu to be transcribed.

The Kali cult towards northern Kerala has different rituals. Dr Chelanat Achuta Menon in his brilliant treatise *The Kali Cult in Malabar* has tried to codify some of the related songs and rituals. The song invoking the goddess in the southern part of the former Malabar district, called 'Pana', which is not composed in the ballad form.   The content of these songs and the mythology around these ritualistic observations show a significant difference.   In the songs and legends prevalent in the north it is only Kali's fight with 'Darika' that is discussed. But the 'Thottampattu' of the south has an additional theme. There Kali appears less divine and the incidents depicted resemble the story of 'Chilapatikaram'.   Kali kills the goldsmith who cheats her husband, in the same way that she has slain Darika. The same lines are repeated with a slight variation of the proper nouns.   This interpolation may be interesting from sociological and historical points of view.   The mythological stories which connect the deities of Madurai and Kodungallur and even the writing of the Tamil epic *Chilapatikaram*—all have an indirect bearing on this pattu.

The 'Thottams' in all these places have not limited themselves to rituals alone. This practice has most probably from its inception, given birth to exciting visual enactment.   In the south it is 'Kali ootu', in Central Kerala it takes the form of revelations ('Velichapadu' or 'Komaram'), and towards the north the most spectacular 'Theyyam'. Kali ootu re-enacts, with the two central characters, the theme of the ballad.   The hunt is performed in the vast area surrounding the temple or

'Kavoo'. The whole story is revealed in theatrical form, with surprising flexibility of the acting area to the very end, when 'Darika' is beheaded. In some places it is called 'Mudiettu and the presentation details vary. The roles are carried by certain persons chosen from particular castes and families and the man who is cast as the 'bhagvati' often grows possessed. The whole show is as exciting as a happening.

The 'Velichapadu' is also possessed and from this state of trance he predicts the future and divines. There is a theatrical element in his appearance and his oracular revelations.

But, 'Theyyam' is not a representative of the Goddess, but the Goddess herself. The presence of the 'Mother' is invoked into the body of the actor by the chanting of *thottams*. Only after that does he become a 'theyyam' (colloquial for 'Deivam' —God). Theyyam is the 'dance of the Gods'. There are 'Theyyams' in praise of various Gods—good and bad and in rare cases heroes like Othenan (the most famous ballad hero). As the drums beat, the singers sing, and the pipers play, the actor priest impersonates these extraordinary divine beings. He becomes possessed. He bestows blessings and makes prophecies. This is a hereditory privilege of the backward communities like 'Mannan', 'Velan', 'Malayan', etc. The spectacle of this traditional ritual is awe-inspiring. 'Theyyam' retains its primitive character and still remains a unique visual experience. The performing and plastic arts of Kerala have much to learn from the make-up, costumes, rythmic moves, instrumental music and the colour of this ritual. In fact, Kathakali has taken many elements from 'Theyyam' and 'Mudiettu' in formulating its histrionic patterns.

Thottam is a very ancient, predominantly indigenous religious ritual which connects one of the most ancient forms of worship with one of the most sophisticated performing arts Kerala has ever produced, and there remains mainly an element in it which could still be creatively used. This is its potential and uniqueness.

3

YATHRAKKALI
Kavalam Narayana Panicker

Yathrakkali is one of the traditional art forms of Kerala which is almost on the verge of extinction. It is known by different names in different places : sanghakkali, sasthrakkali sathrakkali, chathirakkali, sasthrangam, kshetrangam, pannakkali, panayemkali and panayum kaliyum. The same art form is known by different names most likely because its structure has undergone a great deal of change at different places and at different times. The name sanghakkali suggests that large groups of people or sangham participate in this. It is also believed that the word sangham denotes a group of warriors. Tradition has it that the Brahmins, after Parasurama the founder of Kerala, had formed themselves into an order of military discipline under the 64 grammas (villages) of Nambudiri Brahmins.

Some writers hold the view that yathrakkali came to stay in Kerala in commemoration of the victorious march of *yathra* of the meemamsakas to Cheraman Perumal to defeat the Boudhaas. Anyway the word *sangham*, as also the word *yathra* throws considerable light on the mysterious history of Kerala. The available materials used in this art offer further scope for investigation and research into the social matrix of the country in the distant past.

It is commonly believed that yathrakkali took its origin in the Shiva temple at Thrikkariyur. The exponents are chathira nambudiris. They work on the stage as well as in the kitchen, and hence are supposed to occupy the lower rungs among the nambudiris in the social ladder. There were eighteen such groups who were authorised to participate in yathrakkali.

The overall tone of performance is one of social satire although it contains several ritualistic formalities. Each group of players follows its own methods and may not exactly resemble another in all its details. Generally, the play commences with the item *kanamirikkal*. It is an invocation by the group (gana) to Ganapati or the Goddess for the successful performance of the play. The songs may be either prose and verse, some of which are now available in print. The next item is *keli*, which is preceded by a sumptuous feast. As in kathakali, keli is an orchestral performance on percussion instruments, mainly to announce to the village that there will be a performance that night.

This is followed by *arkkal*. The group, after shouting in acclamation, take their seats around a large copper cauldron placed upside down. Beating on it with *thavis*, big coconut shell ladles, they sing in rapture about the Goddess. Two or three of them become "possessed" in the thrill of the rhythm and the dance movement. After the evening prayer, *nalu padam* the most important item in the whole ceremony starts. Four people move in a circle around a country oil lamp, singing hymns about their favourite deities.

The community supper or *athazha sadya* and the verses sung about the dishes or *kari slokos* are popular items and these verses are rendered while the supper is in progress. *Thoni pattu* or *vanchi pattu*, with their boatsongs follow. These songs or quick tempo are meant to remove the fatigue caused by the heavy food and so to enliven the group. Then moves into *Pana*, which is vocal music to the accompaniment of percussion instruments.

From now on the night-long spectacle begins. The entry of Kaimal or Itty Kandappan provides many interesting sequences. *Kurathi Attam* or the gipsy dance, *cheppati vidya* or magic, *viddhi purappad* or the fool's entry, *ayudham eduppu* or wearing of armour, and *vattam iruppu kali* or the entry of character-types belonging to different castes like kongini (Konkani), and pattar (Tamil Brahmin), are some of the items which make this flexible type of drama most interesting and enjoyable.

It is high time that steps are taken to preserve and revitalise this traditional form of performing art. Already an association has started for this purpose at Chottanikara near Cochin.

4

THULLAL—A Visual Art of Kerala

V.S. Sharma

Thullal is a unique visual art of Kerala, with the local colour and stamp of Kerala. It is really a mixture of Malyali classical and the folk theatre. The most highly sophisticated performing arts like Koodiyattom and Kathakali, and the popular forms of folk culture have contributed to the origin of Thullal. The word 'Thullal' has long existed in Dravidian languages with slight alterations in meaning. In Malayalam 'Thullal' is now known as a particular type of dance which was usually perform-ed by men. There are other forms like Kolam Thullal (Dance by men who wear special costumes and masks) and Thumbi Thullal (Dance of the Butterfly). 'Thullal' denotes a particular kind of dance.

It was Kunchan Nampyar, the most popular 18th century poet of Malayalam, who gave shape and substance to the Thullal dance. We are not sure whether Nampyar himself was a Thullal artist or not. He had enough opportunities to witness and draw the contemporary classical art forms as well as the folk forms such as Patayani, during his stay as a court poet of the King Devanarayana of Ambalapuzha. More than 25 years Nampyar spent at Ambalapuzha and this was the period of the growth of his creative genius. The poet could learn from direct experiences and contacts. One legend says that Nampyar composed the first Thullal poems "Kalyana Sowgandhikam Sitankan" as a challenge to a Chakyar who teased him for sleeping during the play of "Mizhavu" for Chakyar kuthu. Next day Chakyar lost his audience as all the people were now attracted to the Thullal performance by Kunchan Nampyar on the other side of the Srikrishna Temple at Ambalapuzha.

We can only say for certain that many aspects of kuthu, kutiyattam, kathakali and patayani are blended in Thullal in different proportions. For example the humorous diction is borrowed from Chakyar kuthu, the music from Kathakali, while the Aharya Abhinaya and Angikabhinaya are according to the classical traditions. The three types of Thullal ottam, sitankan, and parayan are derived from patayani thullal, which is a prominent folk art widely conducted in some of the southern areas of Kerala.

For the Thullal, minimum costumes are used by the artist. Even palm-leaf decorations are used as ornaments by the parayan thullal performer. Ottam thullal is the most refined form of Thullal both visually and in its literature. The poems are composed in Dravidian metres. For the stage presentation, the dancer and two musicians take part. The dancer sings, and dances while the maddala player and the Tala (kaimani) player repeat the sung portion. The song depicts mainly puranic stories taken from the Mahabharata, Bhagavata or Ramayana. In recent times modern poets have chosen contemporary subjects too. The distinctive characteristic of Thullal poetry is that it is satirical. The poem has the colour of contemporary life and the poet criticises everybody without distinction of class or creed. The main story is only a basis for his improvisation and all sorts of human follies and foibles are exposed to laughter through his depiction of classical characters and incidents. For this the poet may create occasions to suit his purpose. For example if he describes the *Swayamvara* of Rukmini, no doubt he will criticise all princes who come in the hope of winning her hand; the poet may even criticise the gods in convenient contexts during the narration of the story.

Literary historians point out that more than 50 Thullal poems are composed by its pioneer, Kunchan Nampyar. He had several followers and even now the Thullal dance is performed occasionally during seasonal festivals in temples. It attracts large audiences, they enjoy it thoroughly, and the poems can stir the public mind effortlessly.

The four types of acting according to the Eastern concept of Natya Sastra—the Angika, Vachika, Aharya and Sattwika—are well blended in Thullal. But at the same time the form is attractive to the common man. As in Kathakali or Kutiyattam, the elements of Thullal are simple and direct. The Mudrabhinaya is not so elaborate as in the classical art forms and the music is easily enjoyable. The Sattwika Abhinaya is very relevant in Thullal but veera, hasya, adbhuta, and raudra predominate. The soft moods are not usually colourfully depicted in Thullal. The dance form as a whole represents vigour and amusement. However, gentle rasas like karuna and srinagara are also not neglected.

Thullal needs no particular stage or curtain. It is presented by three persons. In the 18th and 19th centuries this form had wide popularity in Kerala. During the last few decades its popularity has diminished and Kathakali has gained more attention. Kathakali cannot be as popular or democratic as Thullal. Thullal has the folk touch. One can enjoy Thullal only if one can understand its *vachikabhinaya* (the oral delivery). The merit of Thullal rests more on its 'vachika' than on its other aspects.

At present the art thullal is being taught in the Kerala Kala Mandalam at Cheruthuruthi and sometimes by certain individual masters. Even women study the Thullal dance now. Thullal can claim to reflect life in Kerala. In no other performing art form do we see such pointed social criticism. This art form is masculine and realistic; it instructs audiences at the same time as it delights them.

5

THE SANG OF HARYANA AND ITS FOLK POET LAKHMI CHAND

K.C. Sharma

The history of Haryana can be traced back to the tranquillity of the Vedic times described in the Rig Veda on the lush and grassy banks of the Saraswati. The region passed through centuries of bitter strife, alien domination, physical oppression and migration. Throughout its turbulent history, the people of Haryana have jealously retained their philosophy of life and social virtue, their value systems in the form of folk tales, folk songs and folk theatre.

One technique of preserving and developing folk art forms over centuries has been *Bhajan-upadesh* or religious preaching by the village Brahmins. These visits of specialised preacher-singers from village to village, Ramlila and other folk-theatre forms and various musical gatherings celebrate special ritualistic occasions and collect funds for social services.

The tradition of *Sang* (folk theatre of Haryana) as we find it in its present day form is nearly hundred years old. Earlier, most folk poetry and tales were committed to memory by itinerant bards and recited or narrated to the villagers in this region. Deep Chand was the pioneer *Sangi* or folk poet whose disciple Hardeva was equally popular. Baje Bhagat was the disciple of Hardeva. The thrust of his poetry was mainly devotional and socio-religious. Sangs were used to preach socio-religious values, to entertain and even to increase recruitment for the army as much as to collect funds for various social welfare schemes. Lakhmi Chand is the most outstanding

and most popular Sangi of Haryana. He was the well-known
poet, singer, composer, actor, director, and playwright, all in
one. His plays and poetry encompass different fields of socio-
religious life and in terms of content, style and impact his
poetry can be compared with the works of eminent Sanskrit
poets. However, his poetry was written in dialect tone to his
rural community.

Sang is an open-air folk theatre form with a raised stage.
The musicians sit on the stage itself with *Sarangi*, *Tabla*,
Dholak, *Nagara* and Harmonium. The story reveals itself in a
series of songs. The Sang troupe travels from village to village
and performs mostly during the night. The rural audience
crowd round the stage and often stay the night there not so
much to enjoy the story as to listen to music. The people know
all the stories of the Sang. And though they know the songs
and the music too, they are prepared to listen to a good voice
and a good orchestra. The cast of a Sang hardly ever exceeds
15 to 16, because the stage is usually small and entries are
effected from the centre stage where the orchestra is also
placed. The force of the dances and the strength and pitch of
the songs make it impossible for women to play the female roles
in a Sang.

Lakhmi Chand, the famous folk-poet of Haryana was born
in the village Janti Kalan in the present district of Sonepat.
Lakhmi Chand began his life as a cattle herder at the age of
ten and was associated with a blind itinerant preacher Shri
Man Singh who moved from village to village reciting his own
simple thought-provoking poetry to villagers. One of his songs
runs like this : *"Jagat sei yoh rein ka sapna re"*... or "Life
in this world is but a transitory dream."

Lakhmi Chand was deeply influenced by the blind man's
poetry and his deep-rooted philosophy and accepted him as
his *Guru* or mentor. He was hypnotised by the music and
metaphysic of poetry in dialect; so much so, that he gave up
cattle herding to cook for Sangi Sohan Kundalwala. In Sohan
Kundalwala's group Lakhmi Chand met Dhanwa Meer and
Dhulia Khan, famous Sarangi players who helped him to learn
how to sing and dance. In brief Lakhmi Chand drew poetic
inspiration from Man Singh and learnt the art of acting and

singing from Sohan Kundalwala whose famous folk-plays were *Jani Chor, Chander Kiran, Jamal Sheela* and *Ranjha.* Soon afterwards, Lakhmi Chand began his career as an independent Sangi. To begin with, his poetry reflected adolescent emotions but soon Lakhmi Chand's creative faculties grappled with serious questions of philosophy of life and the theme, the colour and the style of his poetry underwent a significant change. His poetry was a rich expression of the deeper meaning of life in all its manifestations. The folk-tales of Haryana, which were mostly the themes of his plays became alive with colour, grandeur and depth.

The famous Sangs or folk-plays of Lakhmi Chand were *Hur Menoka, Harish Chander Taramati, Nala Damyanti, Satyavan Savitri, Daropti Cheer, Kichak Veerat Parva.* The themes of these plays were based on the episodes from the Ramayana and Mahabharata. His other *Sangs* were *Meera Bai, Padmavat, Noutanki, Jani Chor Seth Tara Chand, Jamal, Raja Bhoj, Sahi Lakar-Hara* and *Heer Ranjha.* In his plays Lakhmi Chand used the simplest and the most effective vocabulary touching different aspects of life. In this limited space it is difficult to assess the versatility of Lakhmi Chand's poetry. We divide his works as a poet into three categories namely, love songs, songs on the philosophy of social life and lastly devotional songs.

Lakhmi Chand's depiction of natural beauty and the depth of human feeling is significant in his play *Seth Tara Chand.* When Seth Tara Chand's deserted son Chandragupt travels on a ship from Singapore with his bride Dharam Malki, Lakhmi Chand describes the ethereal beauty of the bride against the background of the vast ocean :

Byahli bahu na leke chalya chalta karya ya jahaj
Jhama jham ho rhi thi pani pai

When the bridegroom stands on the deck with his bride the whole ocean sparkles with the rich beauty of Dharam Malki and gives the listener the feeling that the moon is rising from the ocean and not from the sky. It is not only physical beauty which Lakhmi Chand's poetry reflects in widest detail but also the grace and expressiveness of human face which moved his poetic imagination in his play Meera Bai. Two sentries from Udaipur who sneak into the zenana garden and see Meera in readiness for a bath in the royal tank, remark :

Teji main sham subah kasia bhan shanti main chandrama kaisi shan.
Nyun ain laikrdva karte suraj bhagwan, aaj chanchak nyun ain aage.

"In Meera's face merges the glow of the setting sun, soothing rays of the winter moon and the softness of rising sun. It appears that the Lord Sun, instead of rising in the horizon has risen from the royal tank reflecting Meera's face".

The rustic similies of Lakhmi Chand are beautifully depicted in his folkplay *Chap Singh.* This describes the sentiments of a woman neighbour of Chap Singh who receives his bride for the first time after marriage :

Koel tain bi mithi lage aisi mahma bani
Kad kee dekhun bat utar dole tain tale durani.

"Her voice sweeter than the koel's, resounds. Oh ! sister-in-law, alight from the palanquin. We are waiting to receive you !"

The episodes and characters in the folk-plays of Lakhmi Chand were taken from Puranic literature and familiar folktales. But these characters become lively with the inspiration and imagination of Lakhmi Chand. The characters convey the richness of social philosophy which the people of Haryana displayed in their day-to-day life. In the folkplay *Tara Chand*, the hero faces bankruptcy and mortgages his son to his friend Mansa Seth with the following advice :

Tara Chand ne saunp diya suta Mansa ki godi main
Mat pita jyuin seva kariye jab ho jya sodhi main.

"Tara Chand leaves his son in the custody of Mansa Seth, recommending his son to respect Mansa Seth and his wife like his own parents, when he becomes adult."

The characters in his Sangs portray faith which the members of the family had in each other and also a rich individualism prevalent in the liberal thinking of those times. In the folkplay *Meera*, Meera's mother appreciates the spiritual depth of her daughter :

Ek thikane man chit karke beti ka biswas dekhya
Mandir nahi diwar andhera Ishwar ka parkas dekhya.

"With concentration I have seen the divine faith in my daughter's eyes. Even without a temple, in darkness her face reflects the divine light."

The sense of duty and loyalty of the soldiers of Haryana has also been portrayed in the folk play *Chap Singh*. Chap Singh was a military leader in Shahjahan's army. He had the occasion to meet his bride for a short while. Lakhmi Chand beautifully depicts the conflict between the hero's sense of duty and love—a conflict which is ultimately resolved in favour of duty :

Chap Singh nai hajjar hona man main darana lagya
Byahi kanhi ka fikar karanh lagya.

"The moment Chap Singh thought of reporting for duty in the *Darbar*, the thought of leaving his wife alone made him sad."

The social respect shown to women and the implicit belief in their loyalty and devotion is depicted in this play. Sher Khan Pathan, the rival of Chap Singh challenges the integrity of Chap Singh's wife and approaches a pimp to seduce her. After much deliberation, the pimp reports :

Kar khamosh hosh kar dil main dubai ga bin pani
Nam lena tain dharti lorje rajputan ki rani.

"Come to your senses, Sher Pathan Khan and stop these character assassinations, forget these awful ideas towards virtuous women. Soldiers' wives are strong enough in character to face these obstacles."

In the folk-play *Puran Mal*, Bhagat Puran gives a steadfast reply to his step-mother who falls in love with her stepson.

Betai upar zulam karai man dekh Ram kai ghar ne
Pati barta ek saar jaanti chhoti badi umar nai.

"Oh mother ! Remember God before casting desirous glances on your son. Devoted women make no distinction between an old or young husband."

Lakhmi Chand's plays elaborate traditional values, implicit responsibilities to self and to society—the values which are being shattered slowly by the impact of modernisation and urbanisation.

Lakhmi Chand will be remembered for his rich love-poems, his vivid depiction of social life and his outstanding poetry of devotional thinking. In the play *Meera Bai*, Meera requests her mother to accompany her to the temple of Lord Krishna in the following lyrical poem :

Mai bi challungi terai saath main ri meri man
Sri Thakurji kai pujan ka ri cha
Jnan rup ka rasta toh lyun main Hari kirtan kar
Daag dil ka dho lyun main raaji ho lyun Shri Krishan ji ke gun ga.

"Mother ! I would also accompany you to the temple of Lord Krishna as it is my joy to be lost in the worship of my beloved Lord. Through the worship of Lord Krishna I would like to find the path of knowledge and by chanting his name I wish to wash away the stains of my heart."

In another devotional song Lakhmi Chand warns the ignorant man lost in the transitory treasures of life :

Man murakh teri aonkh khul gi punji sakal chhali ja gi
Kal rup ki chakki kai manh jyan ki dal ja gi

"Oh ignorant mind ! By the time the dawn awakens you from your life would be trapped between the grinding wheels of death."

In a devotional song attributed to Lord Shiva, Lakhmi Chand says :

Shivji ke gun man kad gavai ga,
Man jya man beiman pachhtavai ga.

"Oh my mind, when would you be lost in the praise of Lord Shiva. Get involved lest you repent."
In yet another bhajan we find :

Krishan Murari mhari bedna nai met
Araj karun sun tharai panyan kai mhain let
Prabhu Kirshan kala ban kyain
Laggo mera hirdai kai mala ban kyain
Pandvan ka rukhala ban kyain
Met di alset.

"O Lord Krishna ! Saviour from sorrows and agonies
Thus, I pray lying at your feet
O Dark Krishna !
Be like the black beads of my necklace
Remaining closer to my heart
Oh the protector of the *Pandavas*
You removed the obstacles in their life."

Lakhmi Chand never demanded money as compensation for his numerous Sang performances and accepted whatever the villagers gave him to support his troupe. But the impact of his Sangs was so great that a large number of villages in present-day Haryana invited him for giving performances for collecting funds for community work and social rehabilitation like digging of ponds and wells, *goushalas* and village schools.

Lakhmi Chand's poetry is the manifestation of the eternal values in aesthetics, art and life. He had been successful in conveying and preserving the traditional values in social life. As such it is the duty of all socially conscious people of Haryana and art-lover of India at large to study, preserve and assimilate the rich tradition of folk-poetry and folk theatre in this age of confusion in modern art forms which has come to an almost deadend.

(In collaboration with D. Mukhopadhyay)

6

JATRA—YESTERDAY AND TODAY

Sharbari Mukherjee

Even today when a Bengali goes to a Jatra performance he says he is going to "listen" to a Jatra and he goes prepared for a four to five hour long experience that will ring in his ears for days to come. The Jatra which was for some decades neglected and almost forgotten is today a very big draw in the urban areas not to speak of rural Bengal where it had never really lost its appeal even at the worst of times. This traditional folk form has held sway over the entire rural population for over four to six centuries and infiltrated into the urban areas when the latter began to develop. In the narrow lanes of Calcutta and other smaller towns Jatra parties mushroomed every now and then with the local talents and later on major Jatra companies were founded in the cities. There has been an intense association with the common people and, therefore, the form has survived the onslaughts of modern age though not without certain constrictions and unhappy mutilations.

The *Jatra* is essentially musical and operatic in form with very distinctive characteristics. It is one of the most well crystallised folk theatres in India reflecting the best of Bengal's folk traditions and literature. It has drawn upon the vast storehouse of material and music from Kathakatha, Kabigan, Panchali, Jhoomur and Keertan to which an additional dimension of classical music was added to contribute to its richness and variety. The dramatic element is equally strong with tremendous communicational potentiality and which to this day successfully projects the social and cultural needs of

Bengali society.   The causes behind the waning of the popularity of Jatra in the latter half of the nineteenth century and
the sudden resurrection after independence in a vastly altered
form demands close examination.   Though quite forceful this
form could not keep up with the changing times and consequent-
ly lagged behind.   Hence today we find that the lapse of time
has left its scars. No amount of conscious striving to pour new
content into the traditional form has revived the Jatra in its
original completeness but the present generation can at least
justifiably claim to be its restorer and feel proud to be able to
use as an instrument of communication a traditional and indigenous form of theatre that our forefather's contemporaries had
rejected for the perhaps more glamorous western stage

It would be necessary at this point to scan the page of
history since no evaluation is valid without a proper historical
perspective.   We must view the present situation as the product of a continuous heritage that was only eclipsed for a
while. Jatra has always been a robust, vigorous and loud
theatre that had, originally, just a string of songs and verses
sprinkled at random to hold them together. The actor still
remains what he was—all fiery and energetic who thumps the
sixteen by sixteen feet square stage with his feet moving about
like a veritable tornado.   And when he stands he plants his
feet firmly on the stage leaning forward like a tilted tower
ready for further action.   The *Pala* or the   written   script provides enough action and excited verbal exchanges to which the
actor adds improvised bits as his mood permits. The night-long
performances are action-packed today as they used to be in the
past—only the duration has been considerably curtailed now.
The origin of this pattern of performance cannot be traced
back to more than five centuries though many a scholar dates it
back to the days of the Natyashastra and some connect it to the
mythico-religious plays introduced in Bengal by Shri Chaitanya
Mahaprabhu after his return from Mathura and which fact
explains the name "Yatra" (pronounced *Jatra* in Bengali) to
stand for Lord Krishna's journey from Vrindavan to Mathura.
For centuries the most popular themes in Jatra were invariably
drawn from the Puranas, the Epics and other miracle plays of
the region that served the purpose of religious instruction and

dissemination of information over and above the entertainment they provided.

Very little is known about the structure and contents of Jatra before the eighteenth century, for there is no written record. More recent history tells us that it was definitely all musical and which facet has given rise to the expression *Pala-gaan* synonymous with Jatra or that which customarily has to be heard. There were morality plays that invariably projected the war between Good and the Evil, and this characteristic has been well preserved as well as utilised for specific ends through the decades. During the struggle for freedom Evil forces were represented by 'white' men in European clothes whose behaviour was in direct contrast to the native in his dhoti. In present times class struggle has been projected in a similar fashion by polarising the two types, the oppressor and the oppressed, to bring out the contrast. Good and Evil have now donned a modern garb and, shorn of the grandeur of myth, look strained, grossly exaggerated and at times ridiculous.

Jatra underwent change in every period thematically and musically but on the whole retained its very special flavour right through. The kind of overacting, heavy make-up and loudness that are its unique features and which endeared it to the masses were not acceptable to the western educated Bengali middle class from among whom came the majority of the intellectuals and social reformers. Thus the first set of conscious changes were brought into Jatra in the nineteenth century. The form fell into disrepute because of the excessive use of the terrors, the horror, and the erotic elements. On one hand Jatra was used as the chief vehicle of communicating patriotic feelings to the masses, on the other there was a strong wave of westernisation that threatened to sweep away the traditions of the people. In 1865 Dinabandhu Mitra wrote his *"Neeldarpan"* which succeeded in arousing public anger against the cruelties of the British masters of indigo plantations and their treatment of the Indian labourers which was acted on stage. The Jatra repertoire had swelled tremendously having included various themes in love, and the historical, social and political life of the people. With the growth in political consciousness political *palas* grew in number on the Jatra stage. However, a counterforce was acting simultaneously at the cultural level. The "picture-frame" stage of the closed theatre of the West soon replaced the open theatre of the masses. Late in the nineteenth century the entire taste of the urban population changed drastically pushing Jatra more and more to the background. It suffered a major set-back.

By then other undesirable elements had surreptitiously crept into Jatra bringing in alterations in its form, content and above all in its music. The monotony of theme, the preponderance of music over action and the scurrility and vulgarity of the comic interludes were among the serious drawbacks which prevented Jatra from developing into a truly national Bengali drama. From sweeping popularity it dropped to a level where only the villagers and the uneducated were forgiven for attending it. The respectable classes rejected it totally. Virility and robustness came to be representative of the low class vulgarities and this rejection pushed Jatra further towards distortions and mutilations. The comic relief of Jatra is usually supplied by a number of farcical episodes introduced almost at regular intervals and are invariably taken from scenes of low life and low manners like the interludes between a sweeper and his wife or a jester and dancing girls and also introduced at this stage characters called *sangs* who stooped down to anything whatsoever to elicit a laugh.

Other structural changes were brought in about the same time. Between the songs and verses, bits of prose and dialogues were introduced. The *Pala* writers became conscious of the fact that their works were not really theatrical in keeping with the then modern stage—a world which was different with its sophisticated realistic writing, characterisation and acting. Another influence was the cinema which gave rise to artistic problems among Jatra actors who were easy victims of the popular film media. Some *Adhikaris* or Jatra managers recruited film extras in their parties particularly in the female role which were traditionally played by male "actresses". The Jatra actors, unlike most other traditional theatre actors in Tamasha or Bhavai are inducted from all walks of life—among farmers, labourers, fishermen, middle-class businessmen etc. —who, but for their talents, usually had no hereditary background or training. Many a famous theatre actor from the city stage or from the films like Ahindra Chaudhury, Teenkori Mukhopadhyay or Phani Ray have acted in Jatras in the early parts of their lives.

This brings one to the question of female impersonation in traditional Jatra. Men have always expertly played the female roles and that seemed the most natural thing to the actors as well as the spectators. It was always the custom. Today although women are accepted in the Jatra they find it difficult to adjust their own 'femininity' to the stylised woman of the Jatra and men are still the best "woman". The male "actress" was trained to speak in a falsetto without sounding harsh whereas a woman's voice would not carry across to a gathering of a few thousand no matter how hard she tried, since microphones are not used in a Jatra performance. The director-producer Surya Dutta of the famous "Natta Company" who has spent 66 years in the Jatra world discussed the aesthetics of acting by saying, "The natural thing is not the natural thing on stage. When a man acts as a woman it becomes art". Some names like Shatadal Rani, Chhabi Rani have become outstanding in the history of Jatra for their exceptional portrayal of female characters. Jatra will never be the same without these "actresses".

It is in the musical aspect that Jatra has seen the most marked changes. Music is the very heart of this theatre and at the beginning there was nothing but music. Bharat Chandra made his greatest contribution to Jatra by composing "Bidya Sundar" in the late eighteenth century which is a major landmark in the development of the operatics of Jatra. The songs have necessarily a strong classical bias if not composed directly on classical melodies. The most popular ragas have always been Bhairavi, Bhairav, Adana, Bageshri and Behag used according to the dominant mood of the situation. The musical compositions found another dimension when around the turn of this century the *Vivek* or conscience was introduced into the format of the Jatra theatrical fibre. The *Vivek* was a singer who used to come on the stage at a particular dramatic moment very much like the Greek Chorus and served the purpose of projecting an extension of the main character himself or herself. The moralising or drawing of an important conclusion from the course of events would be done by the Vivek, often standing on the ramp (gangway) that connects the rectangular stage with the *Saajghar* (green-room, literally decor-room) and for a while all action would be interrupted and suspended. This gave the hero an opportunity to relax which often could also mean taking off his wig, fanning himself vigorously and smoking 'bidis' on the stage often in full view of the spectators. This is because the demand on performer actor of dance, music is so much that he is given enough of rest to perform again. The *Juri* or the "double" who sing "on behalf" is a relatively recent addition which has now been abandoned. They sat in the four corners of the stage, dressed in quaint looking narrow clinging pyjamas, long black tunics and turbans, and sang once in a while addressing the actors, voicing expected reactions of the spectators. They usually helped in prolonging the performances and hence while trimming the Jatra for present day purposes they have been dropped. After a few decades the Vivek acquired some concrete properties and ceased to play the abstract functions it was originally intended for and lost the philosophical transparency. A servant or monk took its place and played the same role. It was dropped too for bringing in a distraction during the performance.

Traditionally the audience sat on all four sides of the slightly raised stage called the *asar* leaving a strip of area for the gangway and the musicians sat on two sides facing each other with the singers (as more and more actors failed to turn out with good voices more singers were needed), the harmonium player, flutist, drummers to which clarionet players and trumpet player were added. *Dohas* from the Kirtan tradition further enriched the musical atmosphere of the Jatra and more of the singing came to be taken up by the professional musicians than the actors themselves. The drums were loud and attracted the villagers from the farthest corners. No marriage or festival would be complete in Bengal village or town without a few nights of Jatra performances.

The second major change came after Independence when as a part of national reawakening the folk forms were revived with great enthusiasm and hope. In keeping with the public's tastes and aspirations and responding to international trends Jatra, with its inborn plasticity, has suffered deliberate sophistication and commercialisation in the hands of modern writers, directors and ambitious Adhikaris. The changing aesthetic scheme has resulted in hybridisation of technique for themes on guerrilla warfare or the life of Ho Chi Minh, inspiring though they may be, has detracted a great deal from the traditional Jatra. Dialogues have now totally replaced the verses and the highly stylised old formal Bengali that had a definite flavour is being rapidly replaced with polished film language. In his "Lenin", actor Shantigopal, otherwise a powerful actor, all but turned the four-sided arena into a theatre stage, a space that is used by the Jatra artiste from every conceivable angle and aspect. The stage area is three dimensional and four sided to the actor and unless it is occupied in a balanced and clever manner as is done by the Jatra actor the effect remains incomplete.

Modern amenities have brightened up the *rangbhumi* or the arena and enchantment has gone out of the satin costumes, silver-paper ornaments and paper swords under glaring electric lights. A cold flat light, naturally makes, archetypal characterisation, movement, ridiculous. Hence the technical sophistication of lighting the stage electrically, exposed the actor, indecently enough. With microphones the full-throated delivery so typical of Jatra has been subdued to a controlled pitch. Gone is the illusory world of make-belief where nothing more than a chair was used as a prop which could stand for a throne, a bathing ghat or a door-step. Refinement has taken the place of authenticity. Film music has monopolised the musical world of Jatra which is a great loss, for the music had a definite character and vivacity which nothing can aspire to replace. One seriously wonders whether one should call this progress. The question is to create a verse-drama that will preserve the old tradition and yet capture the elegance and nuances of modern speech. It has to be at once popular yet elevating for the masses, rural and urban, for the villages are no longer *far* from the cities today. Even when the content is contemporary, Ho Chi Minh for example, the treatment of the subject should be such that the myth pattern is retained in the structure and kept free from hybridisation which often occurs. Realism has never been the aim in Jatra and that its high melodrama is not a handicap but an essential must be understood first.

A powerful and viable form must be restored to its former meaningfulness remembering all the while that they must be purposeful for use in the future. The Jatra has survived the vulgarities of commercialised man and neon lights; and with a little more effort by a few more dedicated souls it will last out the test of time.

7

MASK DANCES OF BENGAL

Asutosh Bhattacharya

Among the various types of mask dances which still exist in Bengal two are very popular—one is known as the *Chhau* and the other as the *Gambhira* dance. They are prevalent in widely separate areas and though both of them are performed on the same occasion, yet they do not seem mutually related to one another.

Chhau is prevalent throughout the district of Purulia which is situated on the western border of West Bengal with Orissa in the south and Bihar to the the west. It is also prevalent in the adjoining areas of the Jhargram subdivision of Midnapore in the south-east and the west of the Kasai river in the Bankura in the north-east. It has crossed the border of West Bengal and entered Seraikella, now in Bihar; towards the south-west and; being patronised by the local royal family, developed to a fine degree though not without the sacrifice of its rural character, in most cases. As a matter of fact, an urbanised form of this dance has developed, with its centre at Seraikella, the border of Bihar, and spread towards the Oriya-speaking areas of Orissa. Therefore, it is sometimes believed that Chhau is a folk-dance of Orissa. But from a study of its rural forms with their accompanying ritual and tradition as it exists in the district of Purulia in West Bengal, it will be apparent that it is a remarkable folk product of Bengal. Chhau is a ritual dance and it is performed in the rural areas of West Bengal in its fundamental ritual character. Therefore an off-season performance of the dance does not represent its true character.

The mask dance known as Gambhira is confined to the district of Maldah, in North Bengal. It has developed an entirely different character. Though the district of Maldah is situated on the western border of West Bengal adjoining the State of Bihar in the west, yet this element of folk-art, which truly represents the character of Bengali culture, has not crossed the border towards Bihar. Probably due to an overwhelming Muslim population in the surrounding areas, this particular form of Hindu ritual dance has not been allowed to spread in any other direction. The case was different with Chhau, surrounded by the Hindu and semi-Hindu population of aboriginal origin. Therefore, unlike the Gambhira it could and did spread in all directions. Gambhira exists as an isolated pocket and as a result it has become stereotyped and devoid of vitality.

Two types of masks are used by the dancers through these two areas. The main ingredient for the masks in Purulia is paper pulp. The masks are therefore, very light in weight and can be used without any effort in the course of a long dance performance. But the masks for Gambhira are made of a special wood which is considered sacred. They are very heavy and difficult to wear during the course of a long dance performance. Great physical effort is necessary on the part of the performers to retain them steadily. As they cover the entire face, including the eyes, the dancers sometimes dance at random, seldom following any rhythm or beat of the drum. The Chhau is largely a group dance, though, very seldom, solo peformances can sometimes be witnessed. But the Gambhira is always solo.

The story of the Ramayana, in particular; the Mahabharata and the other Puranas are represented through Chhau, though in order to give relief to rural listeners, secular legends are sometimes introduced. But in the Gambhira dance there is absolutely no scope for representing any secular incident or a continuous narrative. Only solo dances of characters representing one or other of the Puranic deities are performed to the loud beat of drums. It is believed that in the course of such dance performances, the participant loses his human identity and is animated by 'divine' inspiration. The dancer often grows wild and he dances unrhythmic. Though Chhau is also ritual in character, it can never be wild or unrhythmic at any time.

Both forms of dance—Chhau and Gambhira are ceremonially performed on the occasion of the popular annual Sun festival of Bengal. In both cases it is held mainly on the last day of the Bengali year corresponding to the 13th of April. It is however, continued, in both cases, upto the 13th day of the Bengali month of *Jyestha* (May-June) or the day on which the auspicious event of *Akhsay-tritiya* falls according to the Bengali almanac. The ritual dance carries through a period of one-and-a-half months, to the sowing season of the Bengali cultivators. Therefore, it will be seen that both these performances are integrated into the socio-economic life of the peasants of Bengal, and into the seasonal mythic cycle.

Common Origin

Both these forms of dance being performed on the same occasion e.g., the annual sun-festival, it would appear that both of them originated from a common source, probably with regard to the primitive idea of the movement of the sun in the sky, or control of rainfall by the sun-god, during the period of extreme water scarcity in the summer. Dances are, in a sense, sympathetic magic which help the sun move to produce rainfall.

Over those areas of Bengal where mask dances are not prevalent on this occasion, dances of other types are however, widely distributed. This is the period of the largest dance festivals in Bengal from the popular point of view. The sun-festival, which is held during this occasion, is the national festival of the people of the State, while Durga Puja which is supposed to be the national festival in this area is confined to the upper middle classes. But the sun-festival, during which dances of all sorts are performed throughout the length and breadth of Bengal, east and west, is indeed the national festival, inasmuch as it is prevalent among the people. Almost everywhere, except where there are Chhau and Gambhira, the dancers on this occasion paint their faces instead of making them. The main characters are the great god Shiva and his consort, Parvati.

From an analysis of the rituals it is apparent that Shiva

represents the Sun-god and Parvati, the Earth-goddess. On this occasion the Sun-god Shiva and the Earth-goddess, Parvati, are ceremonially given in marriage. Every year this divine marriage is performed by the peasants of Bengal in the hope of bumper crops during the months to come and dances are held to solemnise the occasion. Therefore, it is essential for the agricultural people to hold dance performances on such a sacred occasion. The pas du deux of characters representing Shiva and Parvati is the main feature of this dance. In the Chhau and Gambhira also, these are the two principal dancers.

Masks and Magic

There are probably two reasons for the adoption of masks on such occasions—one is magical and the other is practical. While its use could be a degeneration of the form of dance held without masks throughout Bengal on such occasions, it is a fact that magicians in primitive society used masks in the course of their magical invocations. This may be a continuation of the same practice. Since the ultimate object of dance during this period in Bengal is to produce rainfall through sympathetic magic, by offering the Earth-goddess in marriage to the Sun-god ceremonially, the idea behind the Chhau and Gambhira dances is apparent.

As far as the practical reason behind the origin of the use of masks in Chhau dance is concerned, there are a number of non-religious folk-dances in the district of Purulia in which no mask is used. Therefore, it may be that with the spread of the influence of Hinduism among the aboriginal and semi aboriginal people, masks representing Hindu mythological characters were introduced, in the form of dances which already existed in a primitive form. This gave authenticity to the mythological characters, deities, the heroes and heroines of the Hindu *Puranas* and the Epics.

The construction of masks is not an easy task, because it implies knowledge of Puranas which may not have developed before the arrival of Hinduism. Therefore, masked dances must have been introduced during the period when the feudal chiefs adopted Hinduism, discarding their animistic religion, in order to establish their superiority of social status as kshatriyas.

If the magical theory of the origin of masks in dances is doubt-ful (though there is very strong ground in its favour), this theory of its origin for practical purposes cannot be altogether discarded.

The Bengal school, popularly known as the Krisnagar school of clay-modelling, in Purulia is very closely followed in the making of masks. As a matter of fact, the Krisnagar school, with its realistic character, became the representative Bengali folk-art since its introduction during the eighteenth century. It seems that it is only after the eighteenth century that the making of masks of the present character was introduced in the Purulia district. Hinduism did not come earlier than this. Certain feudal chiefs of the Purulia district, after adopting Hinduism which made its way there from the western districts of Bengal, seem to have settled a community of clay-modellers under their liberal patronage, for the main purpose of making Hindu images. These subsequently took up the local craft of mask-making.

In a village named Chorda in the Begmandi P.S. of the district of Purulia, live about forty families of such image-makers. They form today, the main group of mask-makers for the district. Patronage of the local feudal chiefs having been lost altogether. They live nowadays on popular patronage alone, but they find it extremely difficult to continue their vocation due to the growing poverty of the people of the area.

The wooden masks for Gambhira are made by carpenters. This is a costly affair because it takes a long time to make the detailed carvings but they can be used for a longer period of time than the masks for the Chhau.

8

THE VEETHI BHAGAVATAM OF ANDHRA

Dr V. Raghavan

Karnatak music and dance still have strong bonds with Andhra. In traditional dance-drama, the Bhagavata Mela Nataka of some of the villages near Tanjore in Tamilnad are an offshoot or a graft from the Kuchupudi Bhagavata plays in Telugu country. Many of the technical terms of Bharata Natya and a considerable part of its compositions—*sabdas*, *varnas* and *padas*—are in Telugu. The Kuchupudi tradition is the best known of Telugu dance-drama forms but this is not the only one. In drama and dance, from most ancient times, as the history of the Dasarupaka and Uparupaka traditions of Sanskrit *Natya Sastra* show, small forms generate major ones and from more complete forms, lesser ones concentrating on select aspects, are secreted and perfected. In Karnataka, where we have the Yakshagana, we also have the form taken from it called *Tala-maddale* in which without roles or make-up, the participants sit down and go through the play orally.

When Kuchupudi Bhagavata attained its high water-mark, it gave birth to a derivative solo performance called the *Veethi Bhagavata* or *Gollakalapa*. The masters of Kuchupudi themselves thought of this new type and it evolved through women-artistes of courtesan families (*Kalavantula*) who were proficient in the solo dance-art of *Nautch*. The Kuchupudi tradition did not permit women to play female roles in its Bhagavata stories and the *Nautch* had its own repertoire of detached pieces and love-songs. By crossing the features of these two, the form named Veethi Bhagavata or Gollakalapa was developed and a

line of capable teachers and accomplished exponents refined it
to a degree acceptable to the connoisseurs. In fact, it became
for a time very popular over a greater part of Andhra.

The credit of discovering the art in its last lingering phase
goes to All India Radio, Vijayawada, and late Sri Y. Satyana-
rayana, who was with that station for some time. Later through
the Music Academy, Madras and the Madras State Sangita
Nataka Sangam, I had the opportunity of bringing it to a wider
public and to the students and lovers of the dance in Madras.
The artiste who expounded the art in Madras was Smt. Anna-
bathula Venkataratnam of Mummidivaram, a symbol of ripe
and masterly exposition, who, after some decades of retirement
due to lack of public appreciation and support, had been per-
suaded to recapture the accomplishment of her younger years.

As already said, it is the *Bhagavatas*, those Brahman scholars learned in Sanskrit and *Natya Sastra*, who were responsible
for originating this form and giving it a shape. Instead of
young boys, courtesans versed in Bharata Natya were absorbed
into the art. Instead of disconnected lyrics, a sustained Bhaga-
vata-theme or episode was substituted. These women-artistes
(*Kalavantula*) had already behind them a heritage of music and
dance and some knowledge of Sanskrit, puranic myths and the
rhetoric of love and *nayika-nayak-bhava*. It was now necessary
only to strengthen their knowledge of Sanskrit and widen their
general acquaintance with the tenets of religion and philosophy.
In fact, if as evolved, this form would shed its dance and gesti-
culations, and follow more strictly the trend of a single puranic
devotional story. It would result in another form, still popular,
active and effective, at least in Tamilnad, the *Hari-katha* or *Kat-
ha-kalakshepa*. In this, as in Veethi Bhagavata there is only one
main exponent, usually male though women are not unknown
accompanied by music and oral exposition. Supported by thematic songs and verses, this presents a devotional doctrine with
illustrative stories of Prahlada, Dhruva etc.

The Veethi Bhagavata has a single female-artiste, the main
dancer; she is supported by a secondary female-artiste. To put
across the ideas more effectively, as much as to entertain,
humour(*hasya rasa*) emerges; and for this a Brahman, in more
or less the *Vidhushaka's* role plays the interlocutor. It is

this dialogue or argument in which the chief lady, representing a milk-maid (*golla*), carries on with the Brahman, that provides the *Kalapam*. The *golla* always scores, she cross-examines the Brahman as to his real brahmanhood and expatiates on what a real Brahman is according to the sastras and under the torrent of her questions and Sanskrit quotations from the sastras, the poor Brahman is left breathless.

The *Vidhushaka*-Brahman may also come off in his role of a comedian and vehicle of wisdom. Wherever a song introduces a character, grandiloquently, the *Vidhushaka*, starts off on a parody of the song, a comic technique which is found in a more sustained manner in the traditional *Koodiyattam* presentations of Sanskrit plays in Kerala. The *Vidhushaka* for instance may begin by parodying the *nayaka* and *nayika*.

The *Vidhushaka* does not involve any new character; the player who began as *Sutradhara* and introduced the performance, himself takes on the *Vidhushaka's* role. He is a versatile and multi-purpose character, the constant companion of the lady and also her chorist. The performance begins as with any traditional dance-drama. A curtain is held by two stagehands and the main character performs behind it, her dance to the entrance-song as sung by the chorist. The classic *ragas* of Karnatak music are used in the songs. The *mridangam* supplies the rhythmic accompaniment. *Jatis* are orally recited and intricate rhythm patterns give the dancer's footwork sufficient scope for artistry. These songs are similar to the *darus* found in the dance-drama compositions and to each of these the *gollabhama* dances. She interprets the theme in the songs closely through abhinaya. The art of *abhinaya* is in full evidence, and by the very nature of the theme, the range of the ideas is wide, and there is greater scope for improvisation and interpretation (*kalpana*). With its elaborate display of *nrtta* and *nrtya*, the Golla-kalapam takes its place among authentic forms of the Bharata Natya arts and possesses adequate potential for skill and beauty of exposition.

The Veethi Bhagavatam when it became popular, was requisitioned for temple festivals, on occasions of marriage and other happy celebrations in the houses of rich patrons.

Among the authors of compositions on *Bhagavata*-stories for this art, and among those who, as *gurus*, trained courtesan dancers as media for presenting this art-form, may be mention- ed Ravuri Kamayya and his brothers Noorayya, Venkayya and Satyamgaru, Vempati, Venkatanarayanagaru, Vedantam Laksh- minarayana Sastri, and Bhagavatulula Dasarathi Ramiah. The brothers trained the Chittazallu family of courtesans and other *Kalavantulus* of note. Over a dozen talented dancers of this class who spread and maintained this art are still remembered.

The Veethi Bhagavatam had to face the same dilemma as other traditional forms of dance and dance-drama in the recent past. It used to be performed for the greater part of the night and a full performance spread over three nights. This length of time is no longer feasible and the same neglect and unhelpful conditions which led to the decay of other traditional dance and dance-drama arts affects this art also. Kuchupudi dance- drama and Bharata Natya have been rehabilitated and it is hope- ed that lovers of art and institutions which have been established in Andhra, as elsewhere, for reviving the local art-forms, will devote their attention and resources to the Veethi Bhagavata, or Bhamakalapa too.

9

MITHILA PAINTINGS

Ratnadhar Jha

The year was 1968, and the "godfather" was Bhaskar Kulkarni, himself a "mystic" artist of some distinction. Way back in 1964 he had come upon Madhubani in one of his frequent wanderings across the countryside. The paintings decorating the doorways and mud walls of the villages of Mithila agitated the fancy of this perceptive artist. In 1968 he organised full-scale exhibitions of these paintings, done on paper by women artists (at his request), in New Delhi and Bombay. The suave, sophisticated art world and the sleek corridors of urban art galleries suddenly found themselves exposed to a folk art that was disarmingly naive in conception but breathtakingly potent in execution.

Coming out of their hibernation in Mithila villages, Mithila paintings, popularly known as Madhubani paintings rocked the national and international art scene simultaneously and brought a visibility to its artists which might well have been the envy of many masters of modern painting. A certain art gallery of Delhi exhibited a choice collection of Madhubani paintings for one whole week which reinforced the critics' belief that the women artists of Mithila can sway uninitiated and sophisticated alike. A critic in a national daily wrote : "In this context it is best to remember that the Primitives and the Innocents in Western modern art owe their inspiration to folk and Negro art. In art the modern and the primitive do meet at a certain point. For proof of it one has only to view the two small exhibits depicting the God Hanuman and Goddess Kali. The whole treatment has a modernistic touch....the colour and linear work is astonishing in its rhythmical patterns and its aesthetic beauty. The big size paintings remind us of the dazzling brightness and colourfulness of Psychedelic and Op art." Mrs Constance Mathew of the Royal Ontario Museum said in a press conference "Madhubani is perhaps one of the most important schools of painting existing today. It would probably become as popular as the primitive Haiti paintings."

Art-dealers responded to the "Madhubani phenomenon" in their characteristic business-like ways. Hardly aware until recently of where exactly the place was situated, they started to view Madhubani paintings through a rain of gold, as soon as they heard the rumblings of its newly acquired fame. They "generously" distributed paints, canvas, brushes and other essentials among the local womenfolk and purchased their paintings at ridiculously low prices.

What is Mithila painting all about ? Is this genuine art or is it just naive drawing by innocent village folk ? Has it got a distinctive folk style ? How far do its idioms and motifs resemble or partake of the larger Indian vocabulary of folk-paintings ? How far has it been determined by its socio-economic and politico-historical forces? Lastly, is it going to withstand the onslaught of feverish commercialisation and so sustain itself in the years to come ? These are questions which have cropped up from time to time in the discussion of this folk art.

In the case of Madhubani two important factors which largely determine the broad outlines of a particular style are : the provenance and the social status of the artists.

Of all the elements in Mithila paintings, perhaps the most intriguing is the mysterious and unobtrusive presence of Tantric symbols. The astrological chart is the basis of some of the many forms of *Aripan*. Though the cult and practice of Tantra could never achieve sacrosanct or acknowledged status in Maithil society, derision of this occult science did not deter its heretic practitioners from making a deep impression on the general consciousness of the people. The Maithil psyche retained a mixture of Tantric exactitude and Brahminical ritual.

Despite the ritualistic and sacrificial superstructure of Hindu society, Tantra has persistently served as one of the most durable popular cults of Indo-Aryan spiritual life. As one of the essential though dormant elements of Mithila painting, Tantra has remained the touch-stone of Mithila's religious, spiritual and mystic libido. One of the most curious and frequent figures of Mithila painting is the serpent. A dual symbol of sex and absolute negativity, the serpent figures in the most unlikely places of the painting. The geometric figures in Mithila painting serve an altogether different purpose. While the circle is the universal egg of creation, the triangle is drawn to accentuate the eternal flow of the three gunas or the three dimensions of Prakriti (Nature)—the sentient, the mutative and the static. The swastika besides being the morning sun symbol may also represent the perpetually belligerent, ever victorious, struggling movement of the spirit towards its supreme goal. Besides these geometric figures, rhythmic figures of six, eight, hundred and thousand-petalled lotuses are drawn in numerous contexts. The petals of the lotus represent the vrittis (tendencies of the mind). The colours of Mithila painting are very much rooted in the interpretation of Tantra, the universe is nothing but a play of colour and sound. By contemplating each specific colour at a time a tantric tries to master the attributes of a particular world.

As with the bulk of India's art heritage, Mithila paintings derive their themes from the tales of the Ramayana, the Mahabharata and the Puranas. The eternal couples—Radha and Krishna, Sita and Ram, Gauri and Shiva,—these are the recurrent themes of Mithila paintings. Besides these religious and mythological depictions, *Kohavar* (the auspicious nuptial chamber) is the single most important subject in which the folk artists celebrate the auspicious occasion of marriage with earthy humour, sympathetic magic and in a joyous mood.

Mithila painting is folk-art form deeply grounded in primitive motifs such as objects connected with sexual organs like bamboo and rings of lotus; fertility symbols like fish, union represented through the turtle and the ardours of love represented by the parrot. The sun and the moon occur recurrently highlighting life and light, motion and warmth : the perceptible rhythms of the known world.

Mithila culture has shown remarkable staying-power against

the vicissitudes of time.   Its isolation and self-containment
nurtured a robust spirit awaiting resurrection. The Vedic,
Buddhist, the Islamic traditions were all absorbed into the
placid waters of its independent yet stubborn existence through
centuries.

Although Madhubani motifs and that strangest of all forms
—the Aripan—are no doubt painted throughout Mithila, their
real home is indisputably, roughly one hundred square miles
radius of Madhubani. This can only be understood in the
light of Mithila's long history. The effects of social upheaval
and political forces may not be readily discernible here, but
Madhubani painting is not altogether innocent of them. The
Maithil psyche—particularly the psyche of its women—is a
typical product of a rigid, conservative social structure.   It
should hardly surprise anyone if the absence of social
themes and political topics might reflect its artists' need to cir-
cumvent the oppressive milieu which they could not otherwise
combat. It is in this sense that Madhubani painting comes
very near to a primitive art and enriches our understanding
both of metaphysical concept and artistic libido.

About the artists themselves, (presently excepting the male
practitioners of this art after its commercialisation) Madhubani
painting may be regarded as the exclusive preserve of women.
This feature is unique. It may explain the Madhubani artists'
predilection for explosive colours, and their use of a limited
palette may unconsciously express repressed desires, emotional
needs and their means to wish-fulfilment.

From birth to burial what is the life of an invisible woman
in an orthodox Maithil home ? How did the women of Mithila
respond to the crisis of vanishing identity in society ?—Maybe
by creating an anti-world negating the limits of time into time-
lessness, Mithila painting is the celebration of recluse habitation
and, in turn, of the void. It may be the obvious response of
a captive spirit to the callings of emancipation from physical
bondage and enforced restraint. The widows who take to
painting are distinctive. The fabric of their highly stylised and
peculiarly vernacular art may be so rooted in the potent despair
of the women of Mithila that it remains an open and somewhat
intriguing question as to what would happen to this folk style

once they are exposed to urban, industrial society and its different norms and privileges. It is a question which confronts the survival and growth of many a folk-art form.

The Mithila range of expression can be roughly classified under four distinct descriptions : (i) Mythological, (ii) Kohavar, (iii) Plants and animals, (iv) Aripan. Anthropomorphic figures of various gods appear to establish the vastness of artist's conception. The eternal coupling of divinity emphasises the dual nature of the central force that keeps the universe intact. Heavily armoured, many-armed Durga is the deification of the Primordial Energy at its fiercest. The black figure of Kali, open-mouthed and bloody-tongued is the representation of the same principle that obliges Shiva to keep his cosmic dance in motion. She is the Prime Mover and also the agent of destruction and dissolution.

The murals of *kohavar*, the innermost auspicious chamber where bride and bridegroom first live and love represent the earthly wit and throbbing passion of Mithila painting. The main figure of the Kohavar is a *Nayana-Jogin* (a woman tantric) at each of the four corners of the room whose main function remains to arouse and aggravate conjugal passion. The snakes remind the newly-wed of vigorous sexuality and the languid creepers vibrate in lasya. Plants and animals generally appear in sympathy, but they are also used as independent themes in for their meaningful associations with some mythological god-head. Each ritual and social event has a set of Aripan, symbolically meaningful in depiction and style. *Swastika Aripan* has been variously interpreted as the symbolic representation of Lord Vishnu who maintains the world and the Maha-Rudra of Shiva. There are six-petalled aripan, eight-petalled aripan, Gavaha Samkranti aripan, Shasthi Pooja Aripan and Aripans relating to love and romance.

An art form which is a part of life and which is practised either for sheer joy or for ritualistic functionalism rarely falls victim to professionalism or intellectualism. Mithila painters never felt the need for naturalistic skill. Concerned with movement and rhythm, devotional elation or inspired vision, they barely observed linear narration. The structural balance of space as found in traditional Mithila painting may be an object lesson to many new painters. No corner of the space is unoccupied or over-emphasised. Compositional unity is achieved through rhythmic studding of characteristic motifs. Mithila painting is an interesting study in harmony. A playful Krishna playing his flute is invaded by tiny flowers like twinkling starlets, languid curls of the stalks of tree, a rhythmic swirl of his loin drapery and an animated wash of matching colour. Mithila artists employ a rich variety of motifs intimately related to the theme and mood of the composition. There is a whole inventory of mystic and religious figures which are both timeless and exact : a perfect harmony between the immediate world and its supernatural counterpart.

Except for the Aripan where the - ground is whitened with rice-emulsion, Mithila iconographics may be best summarised as a riot of colour. In an effort to animate inert space, colours struggle to radiate their incandescence. Movement is achieved through a dramatic juxtaposition of one primary colour against the other and lyricism is achieved by tender contrast.

Jagadamba Devi, a septuagenarian woman artist, and child-widow represents a tradition, a point of view and a highly personalised style that is associated with the Kayastha line of painters from Mithila. Her favourite colours are terracotta and black. Her painting shrouded in dramatic but womb-like mystery. She is one of the oldest members of the present generation of Mithila painters.

More than Jagdamba Devi's intensity of imagination, Sita Devi, the most well-known woman painter of the Brahmin caste, represents the variety of the Mithila school today. While her colours quiver and reflect, as the occasion demands, the line quietly follows—automatically and effortlessly. She is a consummate artist of melody, romance, contrast and occasional violence of colour.

Entirely devoted to line drawing, Matasundari's art is a marvel of concentration, poise and skill. Breaking away from the themes of scriptures and mythological tales Matasundari discovers the world of nature—each point of the space revolving round the other, becomes a splendid spectacle of pauseless trance-propelled cosmic dance. We find in a Kohavar painting

—the self-possessed groom, the stooping bride and a bevy of women in rich costumes. Some of the features are clearly primitive in character and effect. The horny textured style of hair, the pointed sharp nails, and longish ear-lobes, significantly partake of primitive aesthetic.

Mithila painting with its forthright, uninhibited style has arrived like a whiff of fresh air in the presently stagnant world of art. The first dazzle of its meteoric emergence is almost over and let us hope that it is not reduced simply to one of many euphoric crazes in the field of art.

10

DEVNARAYAN KI PAR : A PAINTED FOLK EPIC OF RAJASTHAN

Om Prakash Joshi

Ancient folk tradition may contribute much to the creation of contemporary culture. These traditions are carried in the oral memory through folk songs of each region. The folk epic is one of those unique narrative poems that deals with the adventures of extraordinary people : heroes and gods. The epic songs are traditional, and are handed down orally from generation to generation. The songs are in formulaic and ornamental style, dealing with adventures. Epics are chanted among the group or community which has faith in a particular hero. The narrators use musical instruments while reciting the epic, which may differ from area to area. Here then is a unique example of epic singing from Rajasthan where the narrators use a large painting as the background depicting the incidents of the epic and the narrators also dance along with epic-singing. Thus epic-singing in Rajasthan is truly inter-medial as it involves painting, singing, and dancing.

In Rajasthan the tradition of epic recitation with painting— *Par Banchana* is very popular. The painters who depict these epics live in the district of Bhilwara, situated in the southeastern part of Rajasthan at the foot of the Aravali hills. But most of the epic singers reside in the desert district of Nagor.

Devnarayan, the hero of our epic is the incarnation of god Vishnu. *Par* (like the traditional pata,eg. Yama-Pata, other patas, enshrined in stone on the Sanchi Stupa gateways of Sunga Art) means a linen scroll on which the incidents of epic are painted in five elegant colours. This traditional folk epic is painted and distinguished from literary epics in being anonymous and not attributed to definite authors. The institution of *par Banchana* literally means the reading of *Par*. It is constituted mainly of three groups, *catara*,—the painters, who paint all the epic-incidents on a hand-prepared canvas measuring nearly fifteen metres by one and half metres. The second group is of *bhopa* —bards who carry the painting with them and go from village to village to perform and so earn their livelihood. The third group consists of the spectators who witness the performance and pay the singers in cash and kind, known as *chadhava*. The tradition of epic singing supported by painting has remained a living tradition in Rajasthan during the last six centuries.

The *bhopas* (narrators) sing the epic and also translate it into prose. Generally there are two male *bhopas* who sing, dance and show the painting. In the evening at eight o'clock the *par* is erected with the help of sticks in the centre of the village settlement or the area in which the devotees of Devnarayan reside. The epic is chanted to the accompaniment of a three-stringed instrument known as *jantar*. The chief or fore-singer who dresses in *baga*—red dress, worn particularly for *par* reading, is known as *patavi bhopa*. The supporting singer with a lamp in his hand stands in front of the portion about which the songs and narrations are recited. He is dressed in ordinary dress and as he holds a *diya* (lamp), he is called a *diyala bhopa*. The first singer sings till the third or the fourth foot in the line then the supporting singer joins him and they sing the middle part together. The second-singer sings the line to the end.

Bhopas belong to different castes. A majority of them are *gujars*—an agricultural-cum-pastoral caste to which the hero of the epic also belonged. But there are bhopas amongst the *rajputs*—the warrior caste and *balais*, the untouchables, who traditionally do the work of weaving. All the narrators follow a particular mode of chanting the epic. There may be individual styles of performance but *jantar*, *par* and *baga* along with other elements are inflexible by tradition. The caste of narrators also determines the patrons, audience and the communities where they perform.

The audience is formed of various caste groups. Some

groups are traditional and permanent patrons of the institution of the *par* performance, for instance, gujars are the main patrons of the institution and followers of Devnarayan. Other caste groups are casual patrons and participate in watching the performance and if they like they may offer some money to the particular deity, however there is no compulsion as there is with the *gujar* caste. Bhopas are expected to visit the village of the chief patron who donates the *par* to the bards once in a year.

The reading of the *par* begins in the evening after sunset and the evening meal. The patron or village elders make arrangements for the audience. The audience sit in small clusters facing the painting. Men and women are grouped informally and children jump about here and there. Low caste viewers keep themselves away from the compact clusters of visitors. The performance continues till the late hours of the night or even till the dawn.

The *Patavi-bhopa*—the first singer begins the performance with a short ritual and sings *lurna*—the hymn to *Devnarayan*, the central figure in *par*, sitting on a large serpent and with a lotus flower in his hand. The epic tells the story of twenty-four brothers known as *bagrawats*. Sawai Bhoj, one of the *bagrawat* brothers and father of *Devnarayan* obtains a huge nugget of gold weighing nearly five quintals from Guru Babanath, his spiritual teacher. All the brothers assemble at one place and discuss how to use this fortune. The eldest brother suggests that they should go in for business and thereby increase the wealth. But the others object and one of them, Nevaji suggests that wealth is as ephemeral as the clouds in the sky and that they might as well spend it in enjoyment. Nevaji's suggestion is accepted and the *bagrawats* buy horses and leave for Ran city with their gold. They start drinking; they distribute wine to their horses and to everybody else. The wine flows in drains and reaches the snake king Vasak who holds the earth on his hood. He grows angry and complains to Vishnu about the bad treatment by the *bagrawats*.

God Vishnu then asks the goddess *Chavanda*, to kill the *bagrawats* and have the earth rid of evil. Chavanda takes on the appearance of a princess at *Sawar* town. She is married to the king of Ran city, an old man aged 110 years. However, dissatisfied with marriage, she decides to run away with Sawai Bhoj a young *bagrawat*. She leaves Ran city with Sawai Bhoj helped by *Heerna*—her maid servant. A conflict is inevitable. Jodha and Jagroop—sons of Nevaji are killed in the war with the king of Ran city. Nevaji fights furiously but *Rao* of Ran over-powers the *bagrawats* and all of them are killed in *bharat* —the great war. Devnarayan is born to *Sadumata*, the wife of *Sawai Bhoj* after Bhoj's death.

Devnarayan is the incarnation of Vishnu. Rao of Ran tries to kill him but he is saved by his mother Sadumata and they escape to a distant place. After a few years when Devnarayan grows up as a young boy, he is recognised by his family *Bhat*— the family historian and bard named Chochu. Devnarayan returns to the capital town of Badnor, his father's home, collects other sons of *bagrawat* brothers from different places. The bagrawat sons take a fearful revenge on the Rao of Ran city under the leadership of Devnarayan and recovered all their important losses—Banwali—the famous steed of Bhoj, *Jaya-mangla*, the elephant and cattle from different opponents of the enemy camp.

Devnarayan pardons Rao and is kind to all his people. He is known as a deity, can cure lepers, give vision to the blind, and cure all major diseases including paralysis. There are in-numerable temples of Devnarayan in Rajasthan and other near-by states. Devnarayan's followers and bards sing songs in his praise in temples dedicated to him. Fair and the festival are organised on his birthday which falls on the sixth of the bright fortnight in the month of *Magha—January-February*.

The *par* painters belong to the *chipa* caste of cloth printers. They are engaged traditionally in *par* painting. Only a few families of the Joshi clan among the *chipas* do the work of painting in five towns. The number of active *par* painters are limited to a bare fifteen. The bhopas buy their work and will use them for well on twenty years or more by which time it is torn or destroyed. Thus there is not much demand for the paintings by the Bhopas themselves. The painters have now started painting on small pieces of canvas to be used for deco-ration. These small works are enjoyed by western tourists and as a result are being commercially exported to many countries in bulk.

The epic is painted on a scroll of linen, which is prepared by spreading *kalaph*—a coating of starch mixed with gum. First of all an artist does the *likhai*—a rough drawing in *peela:* light yellow. This is the traditional composition. Then he places *Gahra Peela*—dark yellow, for ornaments, *narangi*—orange, for the body and face, *rata*—red for costumes, *hara*—green for trees and decorative designs, *haramachi*—gray for buildings and lastly *shyahi*—black colour is used to mark the outline of the figures and for the finishing purposes. Artists use one colour at a time for drawing all the seven hundred and fifty figures. These colours are prepared by the artists themselves.

The painter may take twenty to sixty days in painting a large scroll which must pass the test of satisfaction by the narrator bard. The *bhopa* visits the painter's house and follows the tradition of his forefathers for acquiring the *par*. The bhopa is accompanied by the patron who donates and pays for the *par*. After discussion and mutual consultations the price is settled which ranges from $ 100 to $ 150. The patron pays *sai*—some advance money with the order. Sometimes the bhopa stays at the painters house for a month in order to ensure an attractive painting.

The *par* is initiated on *muhurat*—an auspicious day and time at the patron's house, who invites his relatives, caste fellows and elders of the village to participate in ritual, performance and feast that follows the next morning of the first performance. It is an expensive ritual performed for the welfare and prosperity of the family, for protection from fatal diseases, winning court cases and for the protection of his herd of cattle. The name of the patron who donates the painting and the date of *muhurat*, and names of bard as well as painter are inscribed on the central part of the painting.

When the painting grows old and unserviceable it is thrown in the sacred lake of Pushkar, home of Lord Brahma, with appropriate ritual by the *bhopa*, but can never be sold. As god has dwelt in the painting for many years, how can the bhopa-priest sell his temple which may not be cared for or worshipped with the same reverence by the buyer.

There are certain famous painters known for their style and composition. Shri Lal Joshi of Bhilwara town and Durgesh Joshi of Shahpura have won the national awards for their craftsmanship. There are some families of painters at Chittorgarh and Raipur who are also working on folk-paintings. These artists make a living by doing commercial paintings. They have developed double standards, as a result of their art. The paintings prepared for traditional bards are still done in the traditional manner with all the necessary rituals, but the paintings done for tourists do not have any attached rituals, though the content may remain exactly the same.

The painters and Bhopas have kept the traditions of the painted folk epic alive. The vitality and popularity of the *par* reading tradition will keep it intact even with the spread of new means of entertainment. The commercialisation of painters while it is to be deplored has yet helped to keep them in the profession.

11

MARATHI TAMASHA
YESTERDAY AND TODAY

Dhyaneshwar Nadkarni

Although some form or the other of folk theatre has existed
in Maharashtra for the last seven centuries, it is not clear
exactly at what stage the *Tamasha* as we know it today, had its
first distinct beginnings.   The work of the Marathi saint-poets,
between the 13th and the 17th centuries, is replete with references to a variety of forms of folk entertainment. Indeed, saint-
poets like Eknath and Namdev have themselves made extensive
contributions to the verse compositions which were utilised for
this entertainment.

These entertainments were presented by itinerant professional troupes and subsidised by the village authorities.   Members
of certain hereditary trades, such as the barber, the dhobi, the
potter and the oil-miller also annually presented a performance
characterised by song, dance and mimicry.   In what was called
the *khel-tamasha* (*khel*-means 'play'), various roles, both on
and off-stage were carried traditionally by members of particular
professions.   The barber, for instance, would be in charge of
make-up; the butcher, a Muslim, would play the *dholki* (a percussion instrument resembling the *mridangam*); the carpenter
would play the *daf* (a kind of drum) and among those who
supplied verse compositions would be the Brahmins of the
village.

Satire was the most popular form of verse composition. The
form of verse based on any particular satire was called *Bharud*
(which literally means a long-winded tale).   Eknath is noted

for the universality of satire in this genre. His targets were the village *patil* (headman) and his shrewish wife, the grasping money-lender and his wife and diverse other village officials. These *Bharuds* reflected the life of the villages in Maharashtra, four or five centuries ago.

The other form of theatre which inspired the evolution of the Tamasha was called *Lalit*. It presented a number of parts based on village types. Village affairs would be discussed among these characters and in the process, the types would be parodied.

It was during the times of Peshwa rule that these forms gradually culminated in the Tamasha. It was the *shahir* (the composer) who was the proprietor of a Tamasha troupe. He was accompanied by a band of musicians. The instruments traditionally used were the *dholki*, the *daf*, the *ek-tara*, (a stringed instrument with a single string), an iron triangle used to beat out the rhythm, and cymbals. To date, these very musical instruments continue to be used in the Tamasha performance.

Next to the *shahir*, the two most important members of a Tamasha performance were the farceur and the danseuse. There would also be an adolescent boy who imitated the manner of a danseuse, but even in traditional Tamasha these days his tribe has completely disappeared. The danseuse, who was often partnered by junior dancing girls, was accompanied by the singing of the *lavni*. It is the *lavni*—a kind of semi-erotic song full of literary embellishments—which has stood traditionally at the centre of the Tamasha. Maharashtra has produced a number of *shahirs* who have composed *lavnis* which may be called the Marathi equivalent of, say, the Urdu *ghazal*.

In the times of the Peshwas, the Tamasha did not incorporate a play (*wag*) as we have it today. It was only the influence of drama proper, in the latter half of the 19th century, which seems to have encouraged the introduction of a rustic kind of play into the traditional Tamasha. The burden of the Tamasha in the old days rested squarely on the shoulders of the *shahir*, the farceur and the danseuse.

While the *lavni* was designed to carry a subtle, semi-erotic content, there was also another type of verse composition which prevailed in the Tamasha of Peshwa days. This had a decisively

mystic orientation and centred round the alleged dichotomy between Shiva and Shakti. The argument was usually expressed
through a sort of question-and-answer session (*sawaal-jawaab*)
during which intricate conundrums would be posed and answered. Legend has it that the *shahir* of a certain Tamasha
troupe would be obliged to answer them. This verbal tug-of-
war would thus go on, and it is on record that more than one
shahir defeated the danseuses of a rival troupe to become lifetime companions.

This form of musical repartee has long disappeared from
the Tamasha, and with it also all vestiges of mysticism from the
verse compositions used by modern troupes.

The Tamasha during the Peshwa regime in the early 18th
century unfolded itself through five phases. First came the *gan*
which invoked the elephant-headed god Ganpati. Then came
the *gowlan* (which literally means "a milkmaid" but, in the
Tamasha context, grew into a song woven around the theme
of Krishna and the milkmaids). The *gowlan* was presented by
members of the troupe who took the parts of the milkmaids
and Krishna with his 'sidekick' *pendya*. There would also be
the comic character of an elderly "auntie" accompanying the
milkmaids, and just for the fun of it, this would be played by
a male.

In the *gowlan*, the milkmaids going to sell their wares—milk,
curds and *ghee*—in the bazaar of Mathura town are traditionally waylaid by Krishna and his *pendya*. The dialogue which
ensues is replete with subtle ribaldry but it also provides a pretext
for the singing of songs. Today, the original *gowlans* (the songs)
have deteriorated into film songs, atrociously imitated by the
girl dancers. The *gowlans* would be followed by a session of
lavni-singing and of the *sawaal-jawaab*. Of this today we
only have the *lavnis*, much diluted in their musical purity and
shamelessly popular modern lyrics, which are sung in a fairly
crude way.

The last phase was the *mujra*, which consisted of a homage
in verse to noted *shahirs* and saints. The Tamasha today provides few examples of the *mujra*.

The crux of the Tamasha today lies in the *wag* (play). It is
not surprising that traditional troupes should base their plays

on mythological themes. The mythological plot is only a pretext for a mixture of satire, farce and ribaldry. This peculiarly uninhibited ribaldry is essential to the full impact of the Tamasha. Traditionally, the Tamasha would have been performed only in front of a male audience and it is the ribaldry which delights this audience with its cheekiness and inventiveness.

In recent times, there have been attempts to use pseudo-historical and even social themes for the play. The acting of the straight parts is very broad, similar to that seen in the Jatra; but surprisingly, some modern Tamasha troupes, with all their present lack of education, display extremely sophisticated standards of acting.

The proliferation of films in the villages has served to give exaggerated status to the musical aspect of Tamasha. Today we have specific troupes specialising in a session of songs and dances, called the *sangeet baari*. It is customary to see an elderly singer standing near the harmonium player, while her three daughters sing and dance on the stage. The mother has had her day as a dancer and singer in her own right. The art of the Tamasha, whether it be that of the danseuse or of the farceur, passes on from generation to generation within the same family.

The traditional Tamasha troupes have long been performing in village tents and in small, congested theatres in the working class or "red light" areas of the cities. Their economic situation today is precarious, and at least some have not escaped the taint of prostitution on the side. This is a pity because there are Tamasha artistes today who, despite their lack of education, have natural vocal, mimic or choreographic talent. The Maharashtra State Government has failed to do anything specific to keep the art of the Tamasha alive by paying subsidies to leading troupes. All it does is to hold an annual festival, which provides an opportunity for "respected" mixed audiences to witness the traditional art form with all its unchecked, but delicious, ribaldry.

For some years now, the Marathi theatre has seen the evolution of a more sophisticated form of the Tamasha. Dramatists and poets who customarily wrote for an urban, educated audience, wrote Tamasha plays incorporating essential elements of the traditional Tamasha and, in large measure, eschewing the ribaldry. Leading lights of the Marathi theatre such as the humorist P.L. Deshpande, the "rural" short-story writer Vyankatesh Madgulkar and the poet Vasant Bapat were among the first of these "sophisticated" Tamasha writers.

Their Tamasha were heavily oriented towards satirising the post-independence socio-political situation in Maharashtra. Political leaders were favourite targets of this satire, although the plot chosen for the play would be based on a popular folk-tale.

One of the advantages of the Tamasha play is its great flexibility in matters of costume and decor. It rejects the naturalistic frame of the normal, literary theatre. It uses no sets. A king can hold court without the architectural trappings one finds in a historical play. When the king rides a horse he simply mimics the action much as a Kathakali dancer would do in a more refined, stylised way. Change of locale is established by the simple stratagem of the characters going round and round the stage for a minute or so.

If, in the process, unexpected anachronisms may arise, they are very much in the spirit of the Tamasha. For instance, the king may be dressed as if he ruled in another century; but the keepers-of-law in his kingdom will look very much like khaki-clad policemen from the Maharashtrian *mofussil*. The *apsaras* who regale the gods in their heavenly abode will be the same Tamasha danseuses, dressed in their traditional nine-yard *sari*, who have danced the *lavnis* in the part of the performance which has preceded the play.

The farceur (properly called the *songadya*, meaning "player with many faces") has retained his importance in the sophisticated, literary Tamasha. On the Marathi stage today we have a line of talented farceurs including Daha Kondke (who has been schooled by an old-timer of traditional Tamasha such as Dadu Indurikar), Nilu Phule and Raja Mayekar. Kondke can fire off witticisms with a deadpan expression and is an adept at ad-libbing with political material. Nilu Phule, a thin wisp of a man with a nondescript personality, has an inimitable sense of timing and ease of delivery. He can also sink himself into different characters in an unbelievably versatile way. Mayekar is noted for his agility on the stage and his inventive slapstick humour.

A new generation has come to the fore as far as the writing of Tamasha is concerned. Vasant Sabnis, who is both an accomplished *lavni* poet and a dramatist steeped in the traditional virtues of the Tamasha, has staged nearly 500 performances of his Tamasha. Shankar Patil, a leading short-story writer specialising in rural themes, has written popular and satirical Tamasha in quick succession. While the frame of these writers of Tamasha plays is a flexible version of a folk-tale, the content is replete with satire of current affairs. In Patil's plays, for example, the corruption typical of *Panchayat* bosses in Maharashtra has come in for devastating ridicule. It is themes such as these that keep up the wide range of the appeal of the Tamasha. It drives home its point for the villager, and it tickles the fancy of the city-dweller.

The sophisticated Tamasha has imperceptibly but decisively influenced the literary theatre. Some years ago, the leading *avant garde* Marathi playwright, Vijay Tendulkar, in his play, *Sari Ga Sari*, made a brave attempt to put a contemporary situation within the Tamasha frame. If he failed, it was because the plot of the play itself lacked subtlety and was long-winded. It also lacked the key element of a Tamasha: a farceur, who is also in some ways a character akin to the Western Greek Chorus, manipulating the strands of the plot as they unfold from situation to situation.

To make the narrative frame of a play more flexible than allowed by the traditional proscenium stage has always been an attempt of modern Marathi playwrights. Tendulkar has continued with his experimentation in another play, *Zala Anant Hanumant*, using this time the character of a *keertankar* to act as chorus. He has thus taken sustenance from the flexibility of the folk theatre of which the Tamasha alone has been a mildly flourishing form.

A more successful effort is seen in Vyankatesh Madgulkar's recent play, *Pati Gele Ga Kathewadi*. It is a costume comedy based on the type of story one comes across in Boccaccio. A Maratha warrior-husband leaves on a revenue-collection expedition in Kathiawar, loading his wife with impossible tasks designed to test her fidelity. Taking recourse to some picturesque stratagems, which include the seduction of her own husband while being herself disguised as a Kathiawari belle, the lady fulfils all his behests.

Madgulkar has chosen a story which derives much from the Tamasha world of folk-tale and fantasy. He has tried to invest the plot within the narrative frame of the Tamasha. The *shahir* of the Tamasha and the *sutradhara* of the traditional theatre jointly undertake the duties of the chorus. Although this mixing of opposite traditions is not an unqualified success, the core of the play remains a subtle mixture of romance and laughter. The literary merit of this play is, indeed, a cut above that of the modern Tamasha play.

Pursued with a certain amount of intellectual vision, the Tamasha could well be the Marathi theatre's equivalent of the Brechtian play. Except for Madgulkar's play, its current manifestations lack Brecht's poetic fancy although it has the same farcical bent and flexibility of enactment. Also, it must be understood that Brecht was preoccupied with deeper historical issues which affected mankind in all ages. By comparison, the Tamasha is necessarily flippant, comparable to the modern burlesque or cabaret sketch. Without sensitive handling it would have no scope for projecting a tragic vision as does Brecht while still deeply embedded in farce.

Will the traditional Tamasha ever benefit from contact with the urban Tamasha ? This is a moot point, considering that traditional practitioners are still steeped in illiteracy and near-poverty. Recently, during a State-sponsored Tamasha festival, Dadu Indurikar complained that urban Tamasha artistes had grown fat on the toil of the impoverished, traditional Tamasha artiste. Although one can establish only a tenuous causal relationship between the decline of the hereditary Tamasha troupe and the professional popularity of the urban Tamasha, we need to look at men like Indurikar with the sympathy they deserve. But the economic rehabilitation of our Tamasha troupes is a topic about which I have no authority to speak. I can only vaguely visualise some sort of enlightened State support accomplishing the miracle of keeping the traditional Tamasha in Maharashtra alive with all its rugged ribaldry and its delightful lack of self-conscious "sophistication".

12

THE POWADA

Ashok Ranade

The *Powada* of Maharashtra is not really a full-fledged form as with certain other forms of folk music. It has its own musical characteristics ; but its *rasion d'etre* is not exclusively musical. It resembles the ballad and shares with it certain features like a strong narrative element, a certain length, a particular tradition of performance and vocal expression. Like other forms of folk music (for instance the *lavani*, *ovi*, *abhanga* of Maharashtra) the powada has been studied and analysed quite extensively as a literary form. Its metrical peculiarities, its imagery, its social and political content and its other features have also been carefully noted, classified and interpreted.

But there is a yawning gap in these studies. The powada has not yet been examined as a form of musical expression. The powada is always sung and performed and the fact of its being written happens to be a matter of secondary importance. That is why it gives cause for surprise. In fact, it was originally conceived and later preserved as a form to be sung and performed under certain conditions. Therefore, its literary features were determined by its performance-orientation. If we go by the metre employed in the powada the division of time or distribution does not give us an adequate idea of its actual nature. It is the intonation and the consequent contours in the pitch-line which must be taken into account.

There is another reason which prompts an immediate musical examination of the powada. The powada belongs to the

category of those fast-vanishing folk musical forms, which
have been till now quite well-established. There are many
factors that contribute to its gradual disappearance. Every
musical form fulfils certain musical needs and when these needs
are satisfied, the form tends to fall into disuse and ultimately
becomes extinct. This especially applies to musical forms that
are functional in nature. When functional music starts moving
out of the need-based structure of a society, it has either to
enter into the art music of a culture or it has to discover a
function similar to the one it originally had. If it fails in either
of these attempts the form inevitably slides down the memory-
scale of people. The powada is about to do just this. Perhaps
this is inevitable in the cultural dynamics of Maharashtra, so
why should one be nostalgic or romanticise the powada
through artificial stimulation by scholastic and musicological
interest if the form itself is doomed to extinction by the inexo-
rable laws of the interaction of social forces ? However, the
pro-powada argument is not a plea for the preservation or
propagation of the powada as a musical form. What is sugges-
ted is an analysis of its music. Secondly, no science of music
can hope to build up a sound conceptual system unless a
musical analysis of folk forms is carried out. The interaction
of art music and folk music ultimately determines their respective identities. Musical studies of art music tend to be thorough
while folk music forms are, comparatively speaking, neglected.

Whenever a form establishes itself musically, it does so because it successfully answers certain needs important in the field
of performance. How are the tempi and articulation related to
each other ? Does variety in melody reduce the effect or does
repetition make for a concentrated impact ? Does a limited
melody range channelise the attention of the audience more
successfully than a wider range ? Under the circumstances, can
we allow an important musical form to disappear without it
being analysed ? At least in the field of art, tradition is a bul-
wark against pointless duplication and against the disadvanta-
ges of working in isolation. On this account the powada calls
for a deeper study.

The powada belorgs to the category of outdoor music. It is
sung in the open, so the voice **must** necessarily be projected

vigorously. Open-throated or constricted singing but always with a high basic pitch is the rule. The tune ranges mostly in the middle octave and occasionally touches the *Taar Shadja*. On the whole, the tune includes many points (repeatedly used) where the consonants of the words can be conveniently stressed. Throughout the performance voice-production is stressed by the fricative, voiceless H. In view of the greater amount of breath-energy involved in its production and the consequent increase in the 'carrying power' of the word permeated with it, this seems logical. The powada as a form of outdoor music needs a longer reach.

Certain aspects of the tune of a powada are also the result of its outdoor nature. The tune has to be straight and simple. It does not permit decorative effect or tonal nuance. The typical voice-production of powada cannot execute subtleties and ornate designs with ease. In addition, the powada seeks to 'hammer home' a point. In terms of simple content, the praise, that is sung of an individual or event demands the repetition of a name or a theme. The contours caused by an intricate tune tend to distract the attention of the audience from the main theme. Hence the simplicity of the tune.

In addition to this simplicity, the tune has to be more unified. This practically amounts to lack of variety. As the powada has to reach many listeners, and that too, quickly; it tends to prefer a single or at most a limited number of melodic structures and it goes on repeating them. The 'mould' is easily recognised and "known" by audiences. It does not demand any independent attention or special focusing on itself every time it appears. Where a melody or a tune is 'used', it is better to have an easily recognisable tune appearing again and again. But what is noteworthy is that the tune does not become 'dead' despite the repetition. It goes on consistently to suggest a definite tonal pattern in which all auditory content automatically fall in place. The sounds are neatly and quickly organised. What is significant is that when we read the text of a powada, we find the words grammatically and phonetically distorted, they seem to deviate from the familiar norms of linguistic usage. The tune guarantees that we will not feel disturbed by such elements when a powada is actually being sung. It is then that linguistic deviation is successfully received as phonetic rearrangement.

It is in this context that the use of short, four-beat *talas* like *Dhumali Kerwa* for powada-singing becomes significant. Firstly, all patterns of even beats are easier to comprehend. Secondly, the tempo used for powada-singing is so fast that intervening duration between two *Sams* is not long. This means that even if one whole *avartana* (completed *tala*, means cycle) is left unsung or even if one note is prolonged for the duration of a whole *avartana*, the performance does not suffer a break in music. The pauses accentuate the sustained notes. In fact, the literary and musical content of an extended note percolate better due to the unfilled musical spaces. Continuity and significant pauses are so perfectly and effectively balanced in powada-singing that practitioners of art music can learn much from this technique.

On account of this forward moving tempo and refrain, the powada, as a musical form, remains singularly free from emotional associations. It is not bound to those established conventions in art music which seek to build a relation of meaning and music. The *raga-rasa* relationship is not adhered to in the powada. The theme could be Sawai Madhavrao Peshwa's festival, or the Battle of Kharda or the heroic Death of Tanaji, the powada assumes a neutral position in so far as the tune is concerned. Everywhere it is fast, equally monotonous, repetitious and bent on achieving a specific purpose with single-minded attention and economy of effort. This is the reason why its 'tunes' are not set in any of the *ragas*. A powada composer like Shahir Haibat shows close acquaintance with the musicological classification of Hindustani *ragas* and he mentions thirty-six *raginis*. Honaji composes *lavanis* to be sung in regular concerts and he is indirectly responsible for the singing-girls substituting these for musical *khayals* and *tappas*, those established forms of art music. But the powada never strays from its chosen track. A *raga* involves much processing and intricate pattern-weaving which in turn, means a different kind of voice-production and the consequent denial of the open-air, out-door character of the form. With *raga*, the audience-level has to reach a certain degree of sophistication. This militates against the large number and the qualitative homogeneity of the powada audience. The powada with its mass appeal cannot afford this.

All these peculiarities are reflected in the accompaniment provided to powada singers. The *tuntune, daph, zanz* (in reality the *manjiri*) are, in fact, rhythm-instruments. The *daph* and the *zanz* are atonal. They do not have a definite pitch; they do not need any special kind of careful and sensitive tuning, and yet they are capable of reaching a wide range. They do so without dissipating the original sound-energy in any significant degree. The *tuntune*, which on the face of it, appears to be a string instrument is peculiarly uncomplicated. It provides a drone to and around the *tuntune*-player himself and what is even more important, is that it creates rhythmic pulses that have a sharp, metallic quality. So, for all purposes, it is a rhythm instrument.

The vocal accompaniment is equally purposeful. These accompanists pick up the burden of the song with the main singer. The syllables *Ji Ji* are used at convenient and required intervals to show a completion of a song-division. These syllables are sung at *Taar Shadja* by the accompanists. This use of the *Ji Ji* line gives a respite to the main singer, allows the earlier stanza to 'sink in' and yet does not relax the tension already reached. Even the listeners are repeatedly shocked into consciousness by the comparatively sudden use of high-pitched rendering. In addition to this, the repetition and rendering is of syllables which are in themselves meaningless. Thus they do not affect what has already been received as meaningful. They only deepen its significance. The lack of tonal colour and of variety in tune, increases in considerable measure the value of these *Ji Ji's*.

It is also noteworthy that powada-singers perform in a standing position. A schematic presentation of voice-qualities in relation to the demands made on the voice by prose is possible. It will be : Conversation—natural voice; Discourse—official or processed voice; Speech—effective voice. We can have a parallel presentation in the case of a singing voice. It can be : Practice—private voice; Concert—efficient voice; Outdoors—effective voice; the standing position is obviously ideal for throwing the voice. Voice culturists vouch for the scientific value of the standing position. Not too long ago some forms of art music (like the *thumri*) were also rendered in this position.

Any form with outdoor musical content can follow the powada with benefit in matters of rendering, voice-production and rhythmic organisation. For a general audience, listening to a story well told, and briefly commented upon, nothing can be more entertaining than a powada. Musically, it has answered certain problems with definiteness and efficiency. It's traditional association with historical tales should not blind us to its specific musical merits. It is one of those forms which students of art music ought to study with greater attention, and more seriously.

13

MOHINIATTAM

Smt. Kalamandalam Kalyanikutty Amma

Mohiniattam is claimed by the people of Kerala as their own indigenous art but few have shown any deep interest to know something about its true form or origin. There are also quite a few wrong notions about this art form. A few articles have, no doubt, appeared on the subject, but unfortunately instead of throwing light on the situation, these attempts have only obscured our understanding of it.

I had seen it stated in a published article that the dance originated when Vishnu in the guise of Mohini danced before the Asuras to regain the *amrita-kalasa* (ambrosia) taken away by the Asuras. Another article stated that it was the dance of Sri Narayana in the guise of Mohini when He wanted to destroy Bhasmasura. Yet there is nothing in Mohiniattam to substantiate these fantastic theories. Whatever the stories of its origin, it would certainly appear that Mohiniattam is the sister of Bharata Natyam or Dasiattam. There is so much similarity between the two forms. Both must have had their origin in the same source or one must have evolved from the other. In fact, those who are not well acquainted with these two art forms would certainly be led to think that Bharata Natyam and Mohiniattam are one and the same. The *Jatis* have similarity; but the footwork is different. The *mudras* and *bhavabhinaya* in Mohiniattam are as in Kathakali but less sophisticated. The movements of the limbs are extremely graceful and of a very special style. Mohiniattam must have been evolved by a maestro who had a thorough idea of Kathakali

and Dasiattam, or as mentioned earlier, Mohiniattam and
Dasiattam in the early periods must have been one. According
to local tastes, a few differences must have arisen. In this
way, they must have drifted apart from a common source.

Similarities

The items in Dasiattam or Bharata Natyam are in the
following order : (i) *Alarippu*, (ii) *Jatiswaram* (iii) *Sabdam*,
(iv) *Varnam*, (v) *Padam*, (vi) *Tillana and* (vii) *Javali.* In
Mohiniattam the order is (i) *Cholkettu*, (ii) *Jatiswaram* (iii)
Varnam, (iv) *Padam*, (v) *Tillana* and (vi) *Slokam*. The purpose
and meaning of *Alarippu* and *Cholkettu* are the same. The
contents of the items are also the same. In Mohiniattam,
Sabdam is not rendered. May be over time, it must have got
out of system or may be this item, or this rendering may not
have been put into shape. In regard to costume and the
ornaments or jewellery, there is also a close resemblance.

The style in which a 9-yard sari is worn with upper folds
and lower folds, with one end of it gracefully covering the
breast is very attractive and dignified. Only the two sides of
the dancer's waist (*arkkettu*) are exposed. A brief choli is
worn. But it would not have been like it is today exposing
three-fourth of the body. The dancers in both Mohiniattam
and Dasiattam have their hair done in the same way. On both
sides of the head are jewellery representing the sun and the
moon. There are ornaments on the forehead and on the
central line parting the hair. There are flowers on the back
of the hair. All these together create an enchanting effect.
The lotus-style ear ornament is the same in both. While in
Dasiattam the dancer wears the ornaments on the bridge of
the nose, in Mohiniattam the dancer has nose rings on both
the nostrils with a dangling droplet. In Dasiattam, the sari
and the choli are of bright colours, while in Mohiniattam, the
dress is spotless white.

Neglect

We have seen the many similarities between these two art
forms. All the same, today the position and the total image
of Dasiattam and Mohiniattam are vastly different. Dasiattam

has advanced considerably. The image of Dasiattam has undergone change. While it has reached a high pinnacle today, almost exciting envy, it is also a fact that it has lost the extreme beauty of the original movements and the *bhava*. Because of the new acrobatics around *Jatis* very often a *tandava* style creeps in. But it can be stated definitely that very few dance forms have attained such widespread popularity.

In the case of Mohiniattam, the form has remained stagnant for quite some time. It has not progressed from its original position. In the earlier stage both Mohiniattam and Dasiattam were great art forms performed in the premises of the temple. They were pure art offerings performed with great love for God and with hearts filled with *bhakti*. Like the *bhajan* songs rendered in the temples, these dances were unblemished and noble. Even today in the temples of Kerala and Tamilnadu, the statues, (or memorials in stone) of these divine dancers can be seen.

During the reign of the Perumals, Mohiniattam attained popularity in central Kerala. In the sacred premises of the *Kovilakams*, the tinkling of the anklet bells of these dancers merged with the recitations of *slokas* and *kirtans*, the blowing of conches and gongs, and flowed as one stream of dedicated art. Slowly, through the *nattuvnars* (teachers) who had complete control over these *nartakis* and who sought patronage in the lordly manors, many corruptions crept in. The dance, which had a religious purpose, became steadily debased with a certain obscenity introduced to please the worldly and affluent patrons, as in the case of Bharata Natyam. The dance almost became a taboo in refined society. In the case of Dasiattam, the dance was even banned by the authorities. But the art lovers of Tamilnadu redeemed it giving it a new name, and effecting a few changes. The famous Vadivelu brothers revived the art as Bharata Natyam with some new conventions and *bhavas*, and as a result of steady patronage the art has flourished gradually. Though the new form lost the original sweetness of expression (*bhavamadhurya*) of Dasiattam, Bharata Natyam became famous all over India.

But Mohiniattam, like Ahalya with the curse, had to lie low, silent for years and years. It was some thirty or thirtyfive years ago that the kind eyes of Mahakavi Vallathol fell on her. Mahakavi exorcised the curse and bade her rise. But Kerala did not have the good fortune of catching the eye of people like the 'Vadivelu brothers' to hasten and complete the renascence.

Vallathol's effort

It was after a long period of trial that the Mahakavi came across a gifted dancer named Kalyani Amma. Vallathol arranged a private performance for her at Kalamandalam and removing certain seemingly obscene overtones, helped to forge a chaste system. Rabindranath Tagore once saw Kalyani Amma's performance and he registered his appreciation. With the permission of Vallathol, Kalyani Amma was taken to Santiniketan to work at its dance centre. For some time she was also an instructress at the Kalamandalam. In those times, only Srimati Thankamani (Guru Gopinath's wife) learnt Mohiniattam from her. May be brighter days for Mohiniattam were yet to come, for the gifted dancer Thankamani left it altogether. It was only after a few years that some five or six of us began to learn Mohiniattam at the Kalamandalam. By that time Kalyani Amma had passed away. Her Guru, Krishna Panikkar aged 85, taught us. Madhavi Amma also taught us.

In those days, whenever our troupe performed, there was great appreciation for Mohiniattam.

Most of my colleagues and fellow-dancers of that period are happily alive today. A few months before the Mahakavi passed away, he told me that he was sad because he could not bring about a true flowering or renascence of Mohiniattam. "It is your duty now to attempt it. I am saying this, knowing that you are actively performing the art. All those who learned the art along with you have abandoned it. So you must do whatever you can." I feel sorry to admit that I have not been able to fulfil this command of the Mahakavi. I have not succeeded in my efforts.

Shrimati Santa Rao of Bangalore renders Mohiniattam occasionally. It appears she has added a few things to Mohiniattam and omitted quite a few things from the art. She has replaced some enchanting movements of Mohiniattam, with certain gestures derived from 'wrestling'. Therefore, I could not seek a helping hand from her. After we left Kalamandalam, quite a few of our group have learnt Mohiniattam from there. Their guru is Srimati Chinnammu Amma. One does not know how some aspects of Bharata Natyam and Kathakali have got into Mohiniattam. This mixing up is not strictly necessary. There are enough *Varnams*, *Padams* and *Tillanas* in Mohiniattam to be systematised. We invite those who have the mind and readiness to help us in this task. Every region, every country has its love and devotion to the local arts. Mohiniattam belongs to Kerala, and the people should have this spirit. It should not be that we begin to believe in the excellence of our arts only if outsiders praise them !

Need for Diversity

Each art should grow within the framework of its indigenous system. In the process of adulteration, it loses its true and original charm. True diversity arises only if each individual form retains its pristine purity. Without this natural diversity, how could there be scope for appreciation. Take for example, Kaikottikali (*Tiruvatirakali*). Long ago, as in Kathakali, this art too demanded a certain physical discipline (*meyyabhyasam*). Placing the feet at measured distances, bending the knees, with the waist in firm position, and rendering rhythmic movements raising the hands above the shoulders, widening the knees and moving the hands in measured beats, and rendering the *talas* in four *kaalas*—made this a scientific art. Where is the serene beauty of the art as rendered with its original discipline, and its quality as it is indifferently performed today ? The beauty of this group-dance acquired after ten to twelve years of practice can no longer be witnessed today. We should not permit our great inherited arts to degenerate like this ! For instance, some are rendering Mohiniattam with the same costume and *chenda* and *maddalam* as in Kathakali ! Yet some others with their hair rolled up on one side and with any kind of fancy dress, and with *chenda* and *maddalam*, dance Mohiniattam with abandon.

Kathakali as an art is winning the world, drawing adoration from people. Its fame has encompassed the world. But if all its costumes and all its *melas* (orchestration) are adopted for all other arts, it would be sad indeed. The orchestra of Mohiniattam consists of *devavadyas* : *veena, tambura, mridangam, edayka, kuzhittalam* and flute. They should be soft enough to mingle with the *nartaki's* anklet sound (*dhwani*).

(Translated from Malyalam by K. B. Nair)

14

YAKSHAGANA BAYALATA

K.S. Upadhyaya

Yakshagana Bayalata is an exquisite folk dance-drama played mostly in the South and North Kanara districts of Mysore State. The genesis of this folk art is still a matter of controversy, but it can be stated that it has much affinity with the various regional forms of dance-drama performed in India such as the Kathakali of Kerala, the Bhagavatha Mela of Tamilnadu, and Veedhinatakam of Andhra Pradesh.

Yakshagana is known in different parts of Karnatak by different names. While in the plains of North Karnatak area it is termed *Doddaata*, in old Mysore area it is known as *Moodalapaya*. Its more refined form prevalent in the coastal districts of Karnataka is popularly called *Yakshagana*. Akin to Yakshagana, there is another folk art very popular in South Kanara district namely, *Yakshagana Bombeyaata* (Puppet Show). This has also a hoary tradition of over three hundred years.

Expert opinion of scholars on these various forms of popular dance-dramas trace their origin to the Sanskrit dance-drama which was in vogue in India during the 4th century A.D. Dr Ananda Coomaraswamy, renowned critic and research scholar, has opined that ancient Shaivaites were practising a *Natya Shastra* which was in no way inferior to the *Natya Shastra* of Bharata and that the centre of this *Natya Shastra* was the famous Nataraja temple of Chidambaram.

That these dance-dramas were distinctly different from the Sanskrit dramas was apparent. Sanskrit dramas were a combination of prose and poetry in *champu* style and the characters

therein had to learn by rote the dialogue and there were no
dance movements. But in Yakshagana it is different. Yakshagana is essentially a dance-drama with the characters depicting
their roles effectively through dance, keeping step with the
accompanying music.

There is no historical and written evidence to trace the origin
of the name *Yakshagana* given to this form of music. Scholars
have felt that like *Gandharvagana* this form was named *Yakshagana*. *Gandharvagana* became *marg* music while *Yakshagana*
became popular as *desi* music.

Those who specialised in this form of *desi natya shastra*
were known as *yakshas*. They became a community by themselves having taken up this art as a profession. It is rather difficult to prove whether the word *yaksha* was derived from
Sanskrit or was the Sanskritised form of *desi, Jakka*. There is
also a line of argument that *gandharvas* had learnt music from
yakshas and that *Gandharvagana* or *marg* was the more refined
form of *Yakshagana*. Further, Dr Kota Shivarama Karanth
argues that *yakshini* is called in Kannada, *Jakkini*. There is
prevalent in the rural parts of Kanara, worship of a local
deity named *Jakkini* and the worship of this *Jakkini* with music
must have provided the background for the name of the music.
There is also another line of thought that the *Ekkalagana* in
Kannada is solo music.

The Kannada poets, Nagachandra (12th century) and
Rathnakara Varni (16th century), have described a form of
dance-drama, *Ekkalagana (Ekkadiguru)*. The reference obviously
is to Yakshagana. Our ancestors used to call the exponents of
the Yakshagana style of music, *Yakkhadigaru*, the ancient
Andhras called them *jakkulu*, and the stories sung by these
musicians were known as *Jakkulu Katha*. Sarangadeva, an
authority on music in Ancient India recognised *jakka* as a style
of music popular in his time. The only other reference to the
Yakshagana system of music in any of the Sanskrit works on
dance and music is in the *Sangeetha Sudha* of Govinda Dikshi-
tan. He referred to Yakshagana as one of the systems of
music. This work, however, is comparatively of recent date,
having been written only in 1628.

The 9th century Kannada poet-king Nripathunga, in his

Kaviraj-amargalankara has referred to *desi* poetry and mentioned various forms of poetic compositions, *Chathaana*, *Bedande, Baajana*. Scholars have interpreted these forms as different themes of Yakshagana. But there are no written works to prove this theory.

A Telugu work on prosody called *Appakaviyam* mentions that Yakshagana songs are composed in the *ragada* metre, Sarangadeva (13th century A.D.) in his *Sangeetha Rathanakara* describes a metre called *rahadi* and says that it is ideal for *veera rasa*, or war-like emotions. There is no doubt that this *rahadi* is the Kannada *ragale*. While originally this must have been used predominantly in the composition of Yakshagana songs, now other metrical compositions like *bhamini, vaardhakya, kanda, vritta, dwipadi* and *shatpadi* are principally used.

It is quite clear from the writings of the great Kannada poet, Rathnakara Varni (circa 1557 A.D.) who hails from this region that there was in his time a system of dramatic entertainment consisting of music and dance with a hoary tradition of its own. The *bayalata* tradition must have had at least a hundred years' fruitful development before then and the date of its attaining its own distinctive character and the stature of a great form of art must, therefore, be pushed back to about 1450 A.D. Dr Shivaram Karanth cites many authorities to prove that the "Yakshagana" system of music was in vogue earlier still and declares that it has at least a thousand years history behind it. Yakshagana has flourished in the Kanara districts for centuries. One can see its powerful influence still surviving in the rites and rituals and matins and vespers of ancient temples and in the hymnal chorus at old-fashioned weddings.

A matching system of dance also grew up, indigenous in origin, native to the soil, representative of the cultural greatness of *Malenaad* or *Nagarakhanda* as this part of India stretching from Udipi to Gokarna used to be known in those days, owing nothing to Bharata Natyam or Kathakali and drawing its inspiration entirely from the ritualistic dances offered in worship of the snake-god, Naga, propitiated from pre-historic times by the earliest inhabitants of the area. Those who have had the privilege of watching a *Naagamandala*, one of the most remarkable of such propitiatory dances, will be able to appreciate how close the resemblance is and how graceful and various the wavy and serpentine movements characteristic of this dance are.

It is quite natural and understandable that there are several similarities between this kind of dance-drama and the drama traditions of the neighbouring areas. If, however, we examine these different traditions, part by corresponding part, we shall find differences and distinctive peculiarities. Take the system of singing, or the style of dancing, or costumes, or the make-up techniques employed in each and make a comparative study; the individual character of each of these traditions stands out unmistakably. For instance in Yakshagana Bayalata there is dialogue but, the Kathakali, Ottanthullal and Ramanattam traditions employ gesture instead. Kuchipudi is particularly full of these.

It may not be surprising to note that Kuchipudi dance seems to have been conceived from inspiration drawn from Yakshagana dance of Kanara by its founder, Siddhendra Yogi (Siddappa), who, it is said took a twenty-year course of study in Madhwa philosophy and other *shastras* at the feet of His Holiness Sri Narahari Tirtha Swamiji, of Udipi Matha in South Kanara. During his stay in this district, he also received training in *Natya Shastra*. Udipi being the centre of Yakshagana dance form, it may easily be surmised that the *yogi* received training in Yakshagana also and that the later Kuchipudi style which came into vogue in Andhra, was introduced by him on the basis of his training in Yakshagana.

There is a type of drama called Yakshagana in Andhra Pradesh ; at least there was such a thing once. It is reasonable to surmise that long long ago they used to employ the Yakshagana style of music in these dramas.

There is another kind of dance-drama known as Bhagavatha Mela which is now being performed only in Melathoor and its immediate neighbourhood and which has an old tradition. The style of music adopted here is the modern Karnatak music and the dance is excessively influenced by Bharata Natyam.

There is no dance-drama tradition at all in neighbouring Maharashtra and so there is no question of a Maharashtrian influence on Yakshagana. Kathakali of Kerala is no off-shoot of the Ramanattam begun by the King of Kottarakara (who reigned about 1655 A.D.). It is the result of a series of experiments with the Ramanattam system on the lines of Bharata Natyam. Any tyro can see that the dances here which can best be interpreted as speaking through gesture and movement, have had absolutely no influence on Yakshagana.

Kolluru Mukambika temple, founded by Adi Shankaracharya, at the foot of the Kutachadri hills of Western Ghats in the northern part of South Kanara district has been traditionally a famous pilgrimage centre for the people of Kerala, who congregate in large numbers there during Navaratri. It is said that the pilgrims to this temple, which is a home of the Yakshagana folk dance-drama, took with them vivid impressions of this unique form of music and dance and the Raja of Kottarakara who heard these descriptions was influenced to introduce the Kathakali Natya in Kerala subsequently.

The painting of the face in Kathakali follows the famous classification of character into *Satwik*, *Rajasik* and *Tamasik* while in Yakshagana, it is different. It is, therefore, clear that Yakshagana is an art conceived and developed independently down the centuries by the people of the Kanara districts on the west coast of India.

Let us now consider the main features of Yakshagana. Firstly, it is a dance-drama combining dance and music. It must, therefore, have a story, a theme. The story is taken from the Puranas mainly dealing with the ten incarnations of Vishnu and that is why this is otherwise called *Dashavatara Aata*. The theme is the triumph of good over evil, or right over wrong, of the gods over the demons. Each story is in the form of a minor epic containing about two or three hundred stanzas in the various metres mentioned earlier. These are set to music and sung by the *Bhagavatha* to the accompaniment of two percussion instruments called *chande* and *maddale*. The *maddale* is a variation of the *mridanga* but the *chande* or *chande vaadya* is peculiar to Yakshagana and is especially used in warlike scenes and scenes of terror. Each of such stories set to music is called a *prasanga* and there are today about 125 such *prasangas*.

Devidasa, Parthi Subba, Venkata, Nagappaya, Rama Bhatta

and other folk writers have composed a number of well-known
prasangas, influenced as they were by poetical works of
Kannada poets, Kumara Vyasa, Kumara Valmiki and others.
All these writers belonged to the 17th century and after.

So far as the music is concerned, though only a few *ragas*
are at present in vogue, eighty known *ragas* have been identified by experts as having been used. The main feature of
these is their emotional appeal. There are different *ragas* to
express the emotions of anger, heroism, pity, horror, fear, etc.
An 'angry' *raga* accompanied by the frenzied beating of the
chande and the appropriate dance of actor may resemble the
challenging roar of a lion in burst of fury and have a blood-
curdling effect on the spectator. The minimum duration of a
prasanga is about 3 to 4 hours.

Although these *ragas* bear the same names as those in Karnatak music, they are entirely different in the mode and style of
singing. The derivation of the *raga* is so vastly different from
that of Karnatak music that Yakshagana music is distinctly a
separate system altogether.

Desi raga lakshanas have been touched by almost all musi-
cologists. They opine that in *desi* the *panchamasvara* is a little
inferior and that it is a *chaya* of the *marg ragas*. The *lakshanas*
of Yakshagana are referred to in the Kannada *Chandra Prabha
Purana* (11th century). According to it *desi ragas* do not
possess the refinement required to be sung to the accompaniment of the *veena* and other instruments. But this style has
its own refinements. These *ragas* are known as *chaya ragas* according to some old scholars. These are 'Sayam Geya' in the
view of Ahobila and "*Saayanhegiyate Iyam Shadavaa*", says
Sangeetha Saramritakarata. The distinct features of Yakshagana music are that, though the *swara prasthara* may be the
same as either Karnatak or Hindustani style of classical music,
the *gamaka and alapana* style here is unique. We should be
proud that the *suddha* Yakshagana music remains evergreen
only in the Kanara districts.

This system is transmitted by the guru to the disciple, who
has to devote a lifetime of labour in order to master it. As
already noted, the main feature of this system of music is its
emotive power.

War-like emotions are derived by ragas *Ghantarva, Bhairavi, Kambodi* etc. The ragas, *Nilambari, Anandabhairavi, Todi, Saveri, Regupti, Punnaga Thodi, Mohana Kalyani,* etc. depict the emotion of sorrow. *Madhyamavathi, Todi, Arabi, Sri, Shankarabharana,* etc., depict pity. *Nadanamakriya, Mukhari,* etc. excel in the depiction of the terrible and the bizarre, and other like *Mechu, Kore* and *Davalara* also are in vogue. During the course of the entire performance of the one-night session, the *sruti* will have to be altered at least 8 to 10 times.

The second feature of the Yakshagana dance-drama is that there is no premeditated prose dialogue. It is improvised by the actors and is based on the musical stanza sung by the *Bhagavatha.* While the *Bhagavatha* sings a stanza, the actors dance and when he stops singing they interpret the stanza in the form of a dialogue or a monologue as the case may be. Thus each stanza of the *prasanga* is elaborated and expounded by extempore dialogue. It may also be noted in passing that all female roles are played by male actors.

Thirdly, the dance form of the Yakshagana is peculiar to this art. It is more primeval than refined. Like the *ragas*, it highlights primitive human passions and emotions, especially fury and terror. These two emotions are more constantly evoked as the stories deal mostly with battles, scenes of violence and carnage. There is a variety of foot-work and movements which appropriately express these emotions. The actors dance to the music sung by the *Bhagavatha* and to the resounding beat of the *chande.* In Bharata Natya terms, the dance form can be said to be more of the *tandava* variety, although there are *lasya* movements also.

Bharata's *Natyashastra* has in itself various special features of the different dance traditions of this great country, in a more or less codified form. The 108 *karanas*, the 33 *pindi bandhas*, 32 varieties of *charis, niraalamba charis,* 6 *sthanas,* the *prayoga nyayas-Bharatha saathwa, vaarshajanya* and *kaishiki,* while using the weapons, the *atikranta, vichitra, lalithashankara, suchividhdha, dandapada, vihritha, alaatha* and other *mandalas* expounded in jumps, the face-to-face battle movements and other *gati pracharas* are also identified in

Yakshagana by Bharata Natya experts. These features are still preserved in the various Yakshagana troupes here even to this day. Instances like, Gaya on his *gagana sanchara*, Kaurava entering the *dwaipayana sarovara*. Arjuna starting out on the chariot for his *vijaya yatra* in *Ashwamedha Parva*, Kaurava on his *ghoshayaatra* and game-hunting expedition, Sita-Rama-Lakshmana fording the river, Arjuna climbing the Indrakeela mountain, Babhruvahana getting down into the *Patalaloka*, lust-ridden Keechaka entering his sister's *vanithavihara*, the last day's *ratharohana* scene of Karna, who at the same time is grief-stricken at the loss of his son and roused with the revengeful spirit against Partha, depicting the contrary feelings of *veera* and *roudra* and such other scenes which are exhibited in different footwork by the Yakshagana artistes. This will apply also to the *trivida rechakas*. The Yakshagana artistes, it may be noted, did not become adept in the art by a thorough study of the *Shastra*, from books but learnt the art by hereditary talent and also by keen observation and practice.

The theme for the *prasangas* having been drawn from Purana stories, in Yakshagana there is a special feature known as *voddolaga*, which presents the important characters to the audience. There are *voddolagas* both for *nayakas* (heroes) like Rama, Dharmaraja and also for *prathinayakas* (villains) like Kaurava, Ravana and other *rakshasas*. The classical *mudras* and footwork displayed by the important characters during this *voddolaga* scene and partially hidden behind a curtain is something significant, *Shivabhaktas* like Hiranyakasipu, Ravana etc. very effectively display in tune with the tala, the various daily ablutions and *pujas* offered to *sivalinga*. *Hastamudrika* plays a significant role in this type of *abhinaya*. *Shikhara mudra* to denote heroism and authority; *Mrigashirsha* and *kataka mudra* to denote *Danta Dhavana*; *pallava mudra* for *Bhasmadharana*; *pataka mudra* for looking at the mirror; *mushti mudra* for displaying strength, *karatari mukhamudra* to denote assurance of protection, are among the six important *mudras* that could be noticed in the *voddolaga* scene. The various characters push aside the curtain and enter the *rangasthala* (stage) with footwork of the mixed type of *tandava* and *tandava lasya* depending on the character of the hero or villain whom the actor wishes to portray and also to depict the essence of the story. A very special feature of the *voddolaga* dance is the *bidithige* (*chande* beats), which is different for each character who makes his entry into the stage. This feature of *bidithige* helps a spectator to identify the character in *voddolaga*, even from a long distance just by hearing the beats. An experienced artist of Yakshagana who might be adept in the various techniques of the dance-form, learnt either instinctively or by observation, many a times, may not be aware of the names or the characteristic intricacies of the various *mudras*, steps or footwork. They are ignorant of the *lakshanas* or its history.

A very important feature of Yakshagana, however, is the costume and *aaharya abhinaya*—make-up of the actors. It is at once beautiful, colourful, bizzare, as also frightening. The art of facial make-up or *mukha varnik*, as this art is called, has a long tradition. Different characters have a different facial make-up. The most terrifying to behold is that of the *rakshasa* character. The effect of fear and horror instilled in the observer is to be appreciated only by seeing it. Words cannot adequately express the effect of make-up of such characters. Headgear and dress also play a distinct role in the make-up. There are different types of headgear for different characters, such as the hero, a king, a prince, a minister, a *rakshasa*, a *kiratha*, a *gandharva*, etc. The *kore*, turbans of *kiratha-gandharva's* red turban, the impressive *varnike* of Rakshasa, Karna's black turban, the *kedige mundale* (small turbans) of characters like Arjuna, Babhruvahana, Sudhanwa which are prepared afresh on each occasion, beautiful crowns (*mukuta*) of Hamsadhwaja, Kalamlabhoopa, and such other head-gears have resulted in a valuable contribution of Karnataka – like Chalukya and Hoysala *shilpa*—to Indian art and cultural traditions. Dr V. Raghavan, a great authority on Indology has to say : "Yakshagana make-up is decidedly more graceful, richer and more closely related to the ornamentation found in our sculpture than the Kathakali make-up."

A unique feature of the items used in the make-up is that they are made from purely indigenous materials—light wood, paddy stalk, arecanut bark, bamboos, waste jute and cotton, etc. There are different kinds of *bhujakriti*, arm bands, *kataka*,

waist-bands, *virakaccha* etc.   In fact, the make-up is so devised
that characters like Lord Krishna, Arjuna, Babhruvahana
Ravana, etc. can be distinctly identified by their make-up.

Dress is generally of deep colours with patterns consisting
of squares with alternating colours. The most essential feature
of the costume and ornaments is the colour and glitter. The
mere sight of it is thrilling to the spectator who is transported
to the glittering *puranic* world of gods and demon. The Gudi-
gars, a class of craftsmen of South Kanara and Shimoga districts
of Mysore State, have excelled in this art.

The total effect produced by the rousing music of the
Bhagavatha, the rattling beats of the *chande*, the frenzied dance
of the actors and their brilliant costume and colourful make-up
combine to transport the spectator in a rising crescendo of music
and dance to the din of ancient battlefields and deeds of valour.

As the name itself suggests, Yakshagana Bayalata (*bayalu*-
field; *aata*-play), is a play staged in open fields of paddy after
the monsoon when the harvest has been carted home. The
stage—*rangasthala* as it is popularly known—is a square ground
with a bamboo pole stuck in each corner to mark off the outer
edge; its only decoration being bunches of fresh mango leaves,
green and tender, festooned from pole to pole. About 30 to 40
feet from this is the green room, *chowki*, in popular language.
Here, in the blaze of torches, now fast being replaced by petro-
max lights—the characters do the make-up. It is a peculiar
characteristic of Yakshagana Bayalata that each actor acts as
his own make-up man and serves to impart an individualistic
stamp to the traditional pattern of design. The torches and the
brown soil and the deep green vegetation around, canopied over
by the dark blue sky, provide a most enchanting backdrop for
the play.

The play is preceded by a few traditional dances to keep the
audience engaged as well as to allow enough time for make-up.
In fact, the Yakshagana Bayalata is the only traditional dance-
drama which still observes almost all the details given for *poor-
varanga abhinaya* by Bharata in his *Natyashastra*. Here it is called *sabhalakshana*. The first of these dances is the dance of the
Kodangis, or trainees, and begins after sunset. This is followed
by a prayer to Lord Ganesha. After *puja* in the *chowki*, the

man who plays the jester in the drama (*vidushaka*) carries the image of the deity of the *rangasthala* accompanied by the *Bhagavatha* and drummers and offers it ceremonial *arati*. The argument of the drama to be enacted is given at this moment through recitation of one or two brief songs. The stage is then engaged by two small boys made up as cowherds (*Bala Gopaleka*), and they dance for a while, and when they make their exit two female characters come on the stage and do some *lasya* dance.

After these preliminary dances, the *voddolaga* begins. Most of the important characters make their appearance in this scene, but they stand with their backs to the audience and dance behind a curtain which only half reveals them. Female characters do not show themselves in this scene. After the *Nayaka* who gives the *voddologa* finishes his dance along with his retinue and is seated on an improvised dais, the *Bhagavatha* very respectfully elicits a self-introduction of each character as also the background of the story by putting questions.

The stellar role in Yakshagana is known as *Eradane vesha* (second role) because traditionally, *Bhagavatha* plays the first role. Besides this, generally there are five other roles. *Purasha vesha* (hero), *Sthree vesha* (heroine), *Rakshasa vesha* (demons), *Hasya* (jester) and *Moorane vesha* (third or minor roles). All these roles require intense training in dance and diction and background knowledge of the *Puranas*. The training is mostly by observation and by an expert in the art passing it on to someone in the family.

The most important person in the play is the *Bhagavatha*. It is he who runs the whole show. He controls, guides and directs every little thing. He is the *Sutadhara* without whose approval nothing can happen. It is he who sings the songs of *prasanga* and it is on his rendering of them and on his appreciation of the subtleties and conflicts in the play that the success of the show depends. Every character makes obeisance to him on entrance.

The play ends shortly before sunrise, with the rise of the morning star in the distant horizon. The *Bhagavatha* sings the final benediction, *mangala*, offers *aarti* to the gods and returns to the *chowki* for prayer and thanksgiving to Lord Ganesha.

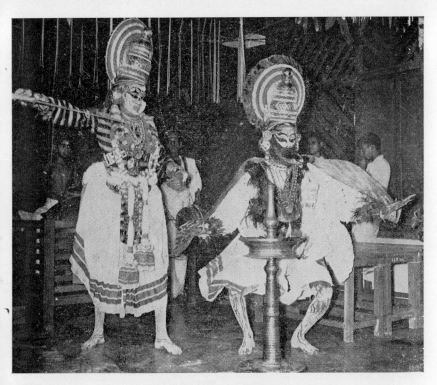

KOODIYATTOM OF KERALA

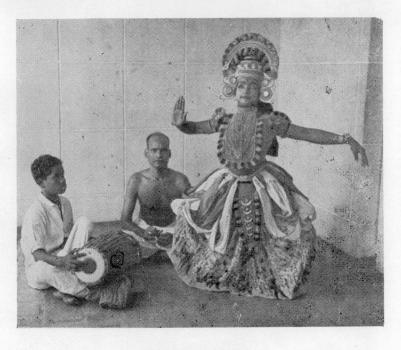

THULLAL OF KERALA

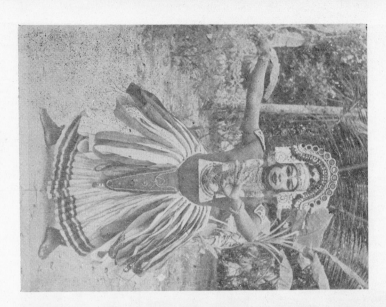

THOTTAM

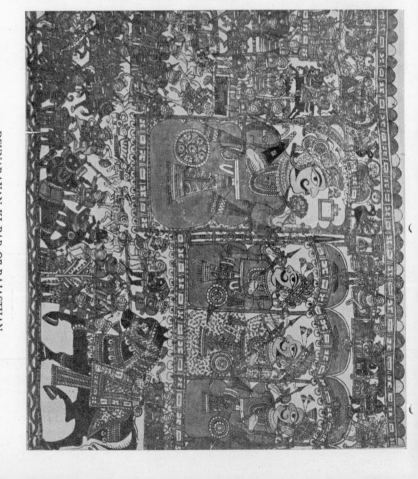

DEVNARAYAN KI PAR OF RAJASTHAN

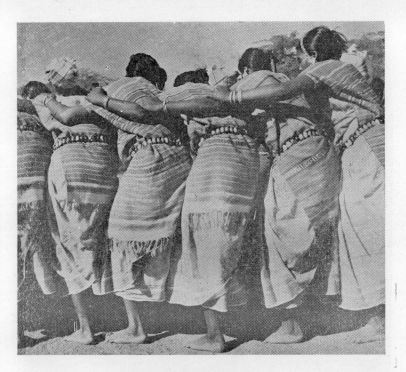

KARAMA DANCE
(*Courtesy* : Sangeet Natak Akademi)

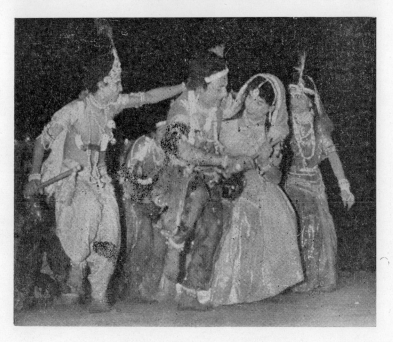

CHHAU DANCE OF MAYURBHANJ

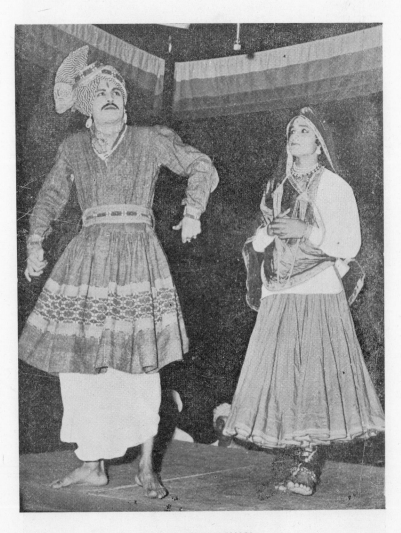

SANG OF HARYANA

Every Yakshagana troupe is generally sponsored or patronised by a temple. Sometimes, to propitiate the deity for begetting a child, in time of trials and stress, devotees offer to organise a drama by the troupe of the temple. A show is organised sometimes by public subscription also. Usually, however, some rich man in the village invites the troupe to perform for the public on his account.

We have quite a large number of these troupes, or *melas*, performing at different places in the two Kanara districts. Only the following, however, have taken pains to keep alive the beauty and grandeur of the traditional style; Mandarthi, Amritheswari, Maranakatte, Kolloor, Perdoor, Kateel and Dharmastala *melas* of South Kanara District and Idagunji, Karkee, Ankole, Kondada Kuli and Gundibail *melas* of North Kanara District.

Those troupes which are mostly maintained by the several temples in the two Kanara Districts are today finding it a strain to maintain the tradition. On an average an artiste in a troupe is paid about Rs 1,500 for the six months he is engaged by the contractor of the *melas* (troupe). This is hardly sufficient for him to maintain himself and a family. And the temples are prevented from spending more on this account by the Mysore Government's Religious Endowment Act. So the artistes are either giving up this profession or turning to troupes who perform solely with an eye to popular appeal.

It is a pity that such a noble art as Yakshagana which, if performed in the traditional way, should give pleasure to and uplift a vast mass of our people, should have come to such a sorry pass. Unless we give some thought to this matter and think of ways to keep the art alive, on the lines of the Kerala Kala Mandalam of Mahakavi Vallathol, we will lose this precious treasure. Kathakali is vigorous and widespread today mainly due to the efforts of Mahakavi Vallathol.

One of the greatest Kannada writers of this century, Dr K. Shivarama Karanth, has done, during the last three decades a tremendous amount of research about Yakshagana and also its revival in its pristine purity. His monumental work on this folk art has received world acclaim. Though he received some help from art lovers in his efforts to sponsor this art in its traditional glory to suit the modern audience, he could but touch the fringe of the problem. He set up a training centre for Yakshagana artistes at Brahmavar with the help of those who were interested in the traditional way. Yet without adequate help such work would be fruitless. The Government or Akademi should help the trainees with attractive stipends in a centre. Yakshagana could also be introduced as a subject in schools like music, Bharata Natyam etc. Research should be conducted to collect more material about this traditional art— about its origin, history and great artistes and composers of Yakshagana *prasangas*. These *prasangas* should be published and preserved for posterity. A Yakshagana Lakshana Granth may be compiled and published. And above all, the still surviving traditional artistes should be encouraged to foster and train young men with subvention for these shows. This is the only way that a future team of artistes could still be found for Yakshagana or else the glamour of the modernisers will kill this traditional art. Fortunately, an intelligent public still looks down upon the cheap modernised shows.

15

ANKIYA NAAT OF ASSAM

Durgadas Mukhopadhyay

"It is natural to long for that which is most beautiful : the gentlest of sound, the most radiant of colours, the sweetest scent, the body which is tender, strong and full of grace." In the period from the fourteenth to the end of the seventeenth century a powerful *bhakti* (enthusiastic and devotional) movement swept across northern and eastern India. After Vaishnavism became popular, folk and traditional art-forms were being increasingly and effectively used for the propagation of religiomystic tenets and beliefs.

Between 1485 A.D., and 1550 A.D., a number of saints, Shankaradeva from Assam, Chaitanyadeva from Bengal, Swami Hari Das probably from Gujarat, Shri Narayan Bhatt from Andhra Pradesh visited from time to time *Braj*, near Mathura, traditionally believed to be the birth-place of Lord Krishna. It is during this period, that a significant development took place in the traditional theatre of India. It was the emergence of *Ankiya Naat* of Assam—the initiation of drama in the field of religion by Shankaradeva. These mythico— religious miracle plays served the purpose of religious instruction and dissemination of information over and above the entertainment they provided. The poet-dramatists of the *Bhakti* movement spoke not to the followers of rigid and determinist Brahminical tradition but to the class of people who believed that the path to salvation lay in devotion to God.

Bhavana is theatrical performance of the Vaishnava *Ankiya Naat*. It is a dance-drama form aimed at propagating Vaishnava tenets and performed in village *Naamghars* (prayer halls) and *Satra* (monastery) premises. The most important *Satras* where Ankiya Naat is still popular and regularly performed are : Baruabati, Baradoba, Dakshinpat, Dihina and Kamala-bari. These plays are based on themes and episodes connected mainly with God Vishnu or his different incarnations especially Krishna and Rama. There are two meanings attached to the name Ankiya Naat. Some hold that these plays are called Ankiya Naat because of the predominance of dance, move-ments of *angas* or limbs etc, in the performance. From the point of view of presentation this view makes sense. Others hold that it is so called owing to its dominating characteristic of having one *Anka* or Act. From the point of view of com-position, this opinion appears to be meaningful.

Ankiya Naat does not strictly conform to any of the types of one-act plays in Sanskrit, namely, *Anka*, *Vithi*, *Bhava* and *Vya-yoga*. Ankiya Naat is dominated by *Bhakti rasa*—the fusion of *Sringara*, *Vatsalya*, *Shanta* and *Veera* rasas. A traditional rhyme points out that a drama is composed of seven rasas. The word *rasa* is used in the sense of "supreme pleasure and in the sense of sportiveness"—*Paramananda-ananga rasa-sagar* and *Srikrishna-jaiche Gokul basika nana binod kautuk rasa ananda karavala*. It also mentions the different objects of different constituents or composite parts thereof ; e.g. *slokas* for the learned, the songs for the Brahmins and other people of the assembly, the *Brajabhasa* for the village people, the masks for the illiterate, the *Gayan-Bayans* for the people having a musical temperament.

In the performance of a Sanskrit play the *Sutradhara* leaves the stage once and for all after the *Nandi* verse is recited while in a *Bhavana* he remains till the end. The *Vidushaka* is an inevitable comic figure in Sanskrit dramas, while it is totally absent in the Ankiya Naat. *Bhavana* resembles the perfor-mance of the old indigenous folk theatre forms like *Oja-pali* and *Dhulia*. In *Oja-pali*, the main character *Oja* sings the story and converses with the chief *Pali*, while other members of the troupe sing and dance. *Dhulia* is a form of group sing-ing and dancing interspersed with comical interludes, either satirical or ribald in nature. Lyricism enhances the dramatic appeal in all these traditional theatre forms. All the players or members of the troupe continue to dance or remain in stance throughout the performance.

Ankiya Naat is lyrical in nature. In the performance there emerges a musical design which reinforces the dramatic sense. There are subtleties of feelings, a depth of perception, and intensity of movements, which music only can express and elaborate. The audience is attracted by the tune, and the emotion and not so much by the plot, the conflict and the climax or the solution of problems. The idea is to create a "poetic fantasia" in the minds of the audience which would convey the ideals interwoven in the play.

Shankardeva (1449-1568 A.D.) was a great Vaishnavite reformer and artist, as well as a versatile scholar and writer. He is the pioneer in the field of Ankiya Naat. His neo-Vaishnavism is centred round the concept of *Eksarania*, which literally means "surrendering to the One". Most of his plays are translations or adaptations from Sanskrit and revolve round the life of Krishna and his manifold acitivities. *Cinna Yatra* (The Yatra through visuals) is believed to be the first play of Shankardeva. His other plays were : *Kaliya Daman* (The subjugation of serpent Kaliya) ; *Patni-Prasad* (The appeasement of the consort) ; *Keli-Gopal* (Gopal at play) ; *Rukmini-Haran* (The abduction of Rukmini) ; *Parijat-Haran* (The taking away of Parijat), and *Sri Rama-Vijay* (Victory of Sri Rama). All these plays were written in *Brajabuli*, the pan-Indian language of Vaishnava saints ideally suited for the expression of spiritual beauty. Amongst all his predecessors and contemporaries, Vidyapati seems to have had some influence upon the language (Brajabuli-Maithili-mixed Assamese) of the plays by Shankardeva.

In the play *Kaliya-Daman*, the high points of dramatic effect consist in the swallowing of the huge conflagration that beset Vrindavana, the twisting of Krishna's body by the serpent Kaliya and the joyful dance of Krishna on the hood of the serpent. The play *Keli-Gopal*, also known as *Raas Krida*, depicts the amorous sports of Krishna with the *gopis*. This is the only play of Shankaradeva, where the erotic sentiment is predominant. This, as a matter of fact is unusual in his cult. Of all his plays this one contains the largest number of songs.

'*Rukmini Haran*' is one of the fulfledged Ankiya Naats of Shankardeva. Here the potentialities of the theme of Rukmini's romance has been fully exploited. The flavour of nationalism adds to the exotic materials of Vaishnava preaching. In *Parijata Haran* humour and satire dominates. The play *Sri Rama-Vijay* depicts the victory of Rama over the princes in winning Sita at the Svayambara ceremony of Mithila. This play is based on the sequence of events as described in the Assamese version of the Ramayana.

Madhavdeva (1489-1596 A.D.) is supposed to have written nine plays. Some of the more important ones are : *Arjuna Bhanjan* (The breaking of the Arjuna tree) ; *Ras Jhumura* (The circular dance) ; *Chor Dhara* (The capture of the thief). His plays do not strictly follow the convention found in the plays of Shankardeva or the works of later writers either.

Gopal Ata (1533-1600 A.D.), the founder of *Kal-Samhati* tenet of the Assamese Vaishnavism was a disciple of Madhavdeva. He wrote *Janma Yatra* (The Yatra on the birth); *Gopi-Uddhav-Samvad* (The message of Uddhav to the Gopis). The other playwrights who enriched the repertoire are : Ram Charan Thakur, Daityari Thakur, and Dvija Bhusan.

Drama is visual poetry (*drisya kavya*) and hence something more than poetry meant to be heard (*sravya kavya*). A drama is able to produce the effect on the observer, the listener and also on the performer. From the point of view of construction, Ankiya Naat may be roughly divided into three parts: 1) the benedictory verses, the conversation of the *Sutradhara*; 2) the story; 3) Mukti-Mangal Bhatima and the colophon, the moral instructions, words of encouragements etc.

Bhavana means 'the performance of an *Ankiya Naat*'. Bhavana is performed in the open air under a wide and high temporary pavilion called *Rabha*. Sometimes it is performed in *Naamghar* or the prayer hall. Bhavana is performed generally on the death anniversaries of the forefathers of the *Adhikar* (director) of a Satra or monastery and sometimes on the death-anniversaries of Shankardeva and Madhavdeva. They are also performed on some Vaishnavite festivals like *Phakua*, *Janmastami* etc. They are also performed for the entertainment of an honoured guest. The Ankiya Naat normally begins at around

9 p.m. and ends at dawn.   In a Bhavana, there are two musical
instruments—the *Midang* or *Khol* (drum with a body of sun-
baked clay, flat ends covered with hide) and *Tal* (cymbal).
Almost all the actors in Bhavana put on conventional dresses.
The *Sutradhara* puts on *ghuri*, the jama and the *pag* (pagri,
turban).   The turban has a grotesque projection in front.   Men
play the female roles and put on a *riha* (piece of cloth) about
five yards in length and one yard in breadth worn above the
waist; from the waist upto the anklet is the *mekhla* (a kind of
skirt).   Three kinds of masks are used : i) of animals such as
Garud, Jatayu; ii) of demons such as Ravana and other
Rakshasas; iii) of buffoons or jesters.   Thick wicks of cotton
soaked in mustard oil rolled at one end of bamboo stick and
when kindled radiates light on all sides.   The ebb and flow of
the flaring torches, correspond to the aesthetic of flamboyant
performance.   A cold flat light would naturally make archetypal characterisation and movements, ridiculous.

The necessary arrangements for the performance being over,
the *Gayan-Bayan* party first appears on the arena with cymbals
and small drums.   They salute the audience by bending their
heads and continue the concert for an hour or so.   The *Adhikar*
enters raising the curtain and takes his raised seat.   With his
permission the *Dhemali* starts, when a large number of drummers play *Khols* in a rhythmic pattern with perfect and easy
synchronisation.   This may last as long as two hours.   The
Sutradhara first recites the *Nandi* verses slowly but distinctly.
The name of the play is announced and he recites a *Bhatima*
or a eulogy of gods, kings etc.   After a little pause the names
of the different roles and events are announced as the players
enter, depart or play their own parts as directed. The Sutradhar
tells the audience to "watch and listen attentively" and to enjoy
the *bhaktirasa* of the play and the audience watch and listen
with the devotional attitude towards Krishna or Rama as a
friend, benefactor, saviour and destroyer of evil.   The prose
dialogues are delivered in a stylised recitative manner.   Here is
a fusion of the diverse elements and influences of poetry, music,
dance, mime, the plastic art and the crafts and tableaux to
create a sublime poetry in space written in a colourful, physical,
earthy language—integrated in a complete whole to transcend

into the realms of spirituality.

At the end of the play the *Mukti-Mangal Bhatima* is recited. After this the priest offers blessings to the performers and the audience. They go ceremonially in procession to replace the icon in its customary sanctuary. Every part of Bhavana is considered divine and sanctified, to arouse love and devotion to the supreme Lord Vishnu.

Assam had preserved Ankiya Naat for centuries. Even today—a time of urban unrest, the Bhavana performance is able to retain its primitive purity and sanctity. Ankiya Naat has survived the vulgarisation and neon lights. With a little more sympathy and patronage from discerning connoisseurs, the tradition could well continue.

16

THE DWINDLING DHRUPAD

Krishna Bisht

Hindustani (as opposed to Carnatic) classical music of to-day is sung in only two forms : Dhrupad (or Dhruvpad) and Khayal; the rest are semi or quasi-classical varieties. Khayal is much in vogue, and at present neither students nor listeners are much interested in the Dhrupad. Not more than half a dozen Dhrupad-singers are in demand at national-level concerts. *Khayal* as the word implies, is imaginative, and it has indeed caught the imagination of the audience as well as the artiste. *Dhrupad*, unquestionably is on the wane. As far back as 1914, the eminent scholar, Fox Strangways said, "...the Dhrupad is somewhat at a discount; it is considered, for instance, unsuitable for public performance."

The word *Dhruv* means 'definite', 'fixed', 'determinate'. Therefore, Dhruvpad means a compositional form having its *padas* or words in a well-knit and definite structure. The common belief about the origin of Dhrupad is that it was de-vised by Raja Man Singh Tomar (15th cent.) of Gwalior. Abul Fazl, the reputed chronicler of Akbar's reign, says about the origin of Dhrupad : "When Man Singh (Tomar) ruled as Raja of Gwalior, with the assistance of Nayak Bakshu, Macchu, and Bhanu, who were the most distinguished musicians of their day, he introduced a popular style of melody which was approv-ed even by the most refined taste." This opinion has been handed down by later Muslim authors. Modern scholars, how-ever, do not accept this theory. Their view, briefly, is that Dhrupad is an evolved form of ancient composed music called

Prabandh, and Raja Man Singh gave it only a fresh impetus.

Bhavabhatta in his Anupa Sangita-ratnakar defines Dhru-pada as follows "Dhrupada is a divine traditional style of sing-ing that shines in the language and literature of the middle country, composed of two or four sentences expressing the emotion of love; it is sung by both men and women. It con-sists of a poem set to the *alapa* of a raga with repetition of final syllables and of groups of syllables conveying different meanings. It has a metrical introduction in two verses, a pre-lude, a chorus, and a final stanza of noble style." (Anupa Sangita-ratnakara) 1 : 65-67.

In passing, it may be mentioned that a Prabandh, by name Dhruv, is found in ancient texts. Dhrupad might have had the elements of ancient Prabandh, but the fact that it was not one of the various types of Prabandhs (Sooda, Alikrama and Viprakeerna) is evident from the fact that Ahobal (early 17th cent.) in his *Sangeet Parijat* describes it under unclassified com-positional forms, and not along with Prabandhs.

Dhrupad, in its infancy, as pointed out by Bhavabhatta (1674-1709), was composed both in the refined Sanskrit and the common regional language of the north. The four move-ments of the ancient Dhrupad were called *Udgraha, Dhruva, Abhoga* and *Antara* after the various parts of the Prabandha, the modern names being *Sthai, Antara, Sanchari* and *Abhog.* From the fifteenth century onwards, Dhrupad became very popular but it was during Akbar's reign (1555-1605) that it reached its pinnacle of glory. Tansen, the immortal celebrity of the Dhrupad style, was Akbar's chief court-musician. Abul Fazl says of him, "A singer like Tansen has not been in India for the last thousand years." Dhrupad was not confined to the precincts of the palace; it was equally popular in temples and hermitages. Swami Haridas, the teacher of Tansen, and Surdas, Govindswami, etc. of the *Ashtachhap* order were all Dhrupad singers of very high calibre.

As an art form grows, it ramifies into various schools and styles. At this time we find the Dhrupad also taking four diff-erent shapes. *Gourari,* the first and foremost school (or *Vani,* as it was called) was founded by Tansen himself, the other three being *Khandar, Dagar* and *Nohar.* Dhrupad continued

to enjoy royal patronage even after Akbar's reign. We have
positive proof of at least Shah Jahan's keen interest in this
majestic compositional form. The emperor had collected all the
genuine Dhrupads composed by Nayak Bakshu. After a careful
selection a thousand of his Dhrupad compositions were compiled to form *Sahasrasa*, i.e. *Sahasra-Rasa*—a thousand essences
or *Hazar Dhrupad*.

Thus we have a clear picture, till the middle of the seventeenth century, of the supremacy of the Dhrupad above other
musical forms. A number of Dhrupad compositions of this
period by great masters like Nayak Bakshu, Swami Haridas,
Miya Tansen, and Nayak Baiju have come down to us. But
when the question of their rendition arises, we are quite at sea,
because there is no record of their notations.

Evidently, the Dhrupad style of singing had developed to
its utmost during the eighteenth century. At this time there
appeared a genius, Nyamat Khan, better known by his pen-
name (incorporated in his compositions), *Sadaarang*. To him
is ascribed the propagation of the Khayal style in general, and
the innovation of the *Vilambit* (slow tempo) style in particular.
He was the composer of the numerous Khayals that are sung
and highly appreciated even today. A descendant of Tansen
himself, he personally avoided the practice of Khayal but
taught it, so tradition goes, to two talented beggar-boys of the
lowest caste. These prodigies grew up to be such masters of the
art of Khayal-singing as to have quite a large following.

For some time Khayal and Dhrupad were equally popular
and there was no conflict between them. But while Khayal
flowed on to become a wider stream, the Dhrupad became
stagnant. From time to time new techniques have been added
to enrich the Khayal style. The creative genius of some of its
masters has made such a beautiful bouquet of it that younger
generations have been drawn to it. It is only natural that the
votaries of the Dhrupad have been far outnumbered by those
of the Khayal.

At this point it would not be uncalled for to assess the
causes of the decreasing popularity of Dhrupad. Some say that
it is because of the degeneration of its poetic aspect while some
others believe that it failed beyond a certain point to convey the

Nava-rasas (the essence of the nine emotive states).   As to poetic content it is quite evident that in Hindustani classical music, poetry is no more than a conduit for music itself. The conduit must be sound, but it is the fluid that really matters. The soul of our music is the *Raga*, and the endeavour of the artiste is to conjure up the picture of the raga, with all its subtle nuances.   It remains an open question whether poetic emotions have any relevance in the context of our classical music, which tends to be 'absolute' rather than applied.

Dhrupad had lost its charm in my opinion because it had become stereotyped. We might say it was almost, moribund. In olden times, due importance was attached to the melodic content. Later on, too much stress was laid on the rhythmic patterns or *Layakari* which tended to degenerate to mere acrobatics. Secondly, the Khayal style incorporates all that has worth in the Dhrupad. Over and above that, it has much more that the Dhrupad does not have. The grace-notes, the intermediary notes, notes in quick succession, and above all, its musical 'licence' were beyond the ken of the Dhrupad-singer. And it is these that have appealed to and converted the succeeding generations.

As to the question of the revival of the Dhrupad; well, when the Khayal has all the niceties of the Dhrupad in addition to its own, naturally many are of the opinion that the question hardly arises. At the same time this pristine vocal art form must be preserved as an entity for academic interest. It should be taught so that the novice may have better command over the rhythm. Further, we may refer to the old Dhrupad compositions for the original and pure form of a Raga as we refer to a gospel as the root from which the flower sprung.

17

GOTIPUA DANCERS OF ORISSA

Sunil Kothari

Gotipua is the name given to a class of young male dancers
in Orissa who, dressed as girls, perform the traditional classical
Odissi dance. These young acolyte dancers have been, albeit unconsciously, of great service to the continuation of the tradition
thus in a sense, making possible the revival of the classical
Odissi style in its present form. It is interesting to learn that
some of the prominent Odissi gurus of today were Gotipua
dancers in their youth.

It is believed that this tradition came into being at the time
of the great saint and singer Chaitanya. Chaitanya's religious
discourses greatly influenced the masses. Vaishnavism spread
all over Orissa during the reign of King Purushottam Deva.
In 1447 A.D. Purushottam Deva's son, Prataprudra Deva,
was ruling over Orissa. He was a devout Vaishnava king and
ordered that only the *Gita Govind* text should be sung in the
temple of Jagannath at Puri. It was Ramananda Pattanaik,
his minister, who was mainly responsible for this measure. The
minister had given up his governorship of Rajahamundry after
he came in close contact with Chaitanya. The saint had
changed the course of his life. Pattanaik then devoted the rest
of his life in the service of Lord Jagannath and later came to
be known as Ramananda Raya.

Sakhi Bhava

Vaishnavism brought in its wake the cult of *Sakhi Bhava*,
the religious belief propounding that God could be approached

only through ecstatic devotion as in the manner of the *gopis* who worshipped Lord Krishna. The story of the preacher Gonsaiji and his encounter with the Vaishnava saint, Meera, is often quoted to illustrate the cardinal belief of this cult in which the Lord alone is *Purusha* (male), and all devotees *gopis*. Gonsaiji had taken so strict a vow of celibacy that he would not look at the face of any woman. If he had to meet a woman, he could only do so with a screen between them. When he learnt that Meera had arrived in Vraja, he went to meet her, but was careful to keep the screen between them. Meera reminded him of the cardinal principle of the Sakhi cult and that she believed there was only one *Purusha* in Vraja—the land of the *gopis*. She maintained that if Gonsaiji had remained *Purusha* in spite of staying in Vraja, his *bhakti* (devotion) must have made him oblivious of the fact that Lord Krishna alone is *Purusha*. On hearing these words of sarcasm from Meera, Gonsaiji realised his folly and touched the feet of Meera.

Ramananda Raya was a devout Vaishnava of this extreme cult and encouraged worship according to *Sakhi Bhava*. It was he who introduced the custom of the temple dances being performed by boys dressed as girls and not by women, as was the custom elsewhere.

Seven Streets, Akhadas, Gymnasia

Such were the origins of Gotipua dancers but historically speaking Gotipuas as an established class only came into existence during the time of the Bhoi King, Ramachandra Deva in 1600 A.D. almost two hundred years later. Ramachandra Deva was a great devotee of Lord Jagannath and personally supervised the rituals connected with the temple. He considered it his prime duty to protect the temple and the town from intruders and regulated the rituals of *sevayatas*, the class of priests performing *seva* or services in the temple. He built, near the temple, seven streets for these *sevayatas*. There were several categories among the priesthood of which one was that of the Gotipuas.

Ramachandra Deva's interest in physical culture resulted in the establishment of gymnasia in several parts of the town. These gymnasia were like club—*akhadas*—which also became the centre of cultural activities. It was in these *akhadas* that Gotipua artistes were taught dancing. Several Gotipua dancers were attached to each *akhada*, and hence the name *Akhada Pila* for Gotipua dancers. To this day there is an unbroken tradition of *Akhada Pila* belonging to professional Gotipua troupes. Generally such groups are conducted by a particular guru.

Arduous Training

The training in physical culture and dancing for the chosen boys begins at the age of seven and continues till the approach of adolescence when the boys lose their delicate appearance. Generally, they do not perform as Gotipuas after eighteen but they then become conductors or teachers and continue teaching Odissi dance. The young boys are taught various exercises and acrobatics, their bodies being trained through difficult physical disciplines. The training is rounded off with music, singing and the playing of drums.

An essential feature of their dancing is the singing which accompanies the dance. Hence great emphasis is placed on the cultivation of breath control, as singing while dancing simultaneously, is very strenuous. Nowadays, however, very few of the boys sing while they dance.

A remarkable feature of their dancing is the use of several *bandhas*—acrobatic feats—which are now not performed by Odissi dancers though they are mentioned in various palm-leaf manuscripts pertaining to dance. Some of the *karanas* mentioned in Bharata's *Natyashastra* are thus found in vogue in Odissi dance. Thus, barring these *bandhas* their repertoire is the same as in Odissi dance, making use of various *pada bhedas*, *bhangis*, *beli hastas* etc.

It is necessary to remember that it was with the advent of the Gotipua dancer that Odissi dance came out of the temple precincts and started being performed in public. If we are fortunate enough to see Odissi as a part of the repertoire of present day dancers, it is largely due to these acolytes who carried on the art and preserved the tradition.

Festivals and Fairs

Two religious festivals of importance are linked with the traditional Gotipua dance which can be witnessed on these occasions in Orissa. One is the *Chandan Jatra* and the other, *Jhoolan Jatra*. Besides these two festivals they perform at several social gatherings. On the occasion of *Chandan Jatra* the Gotipuas give a performance on water, on the *chappo* or boat at the time the Lord is taken out in procession to *Chandan Pokhri* or the tank—for an immersion in sandal-paste after which commences a ceremonial boat ride. *Chandan Jatra* begins on the third day of *Vaisakh* or *Akshya Tritiya* (May) and continues for twenty-one days. Each night there are orders from the officiating priest of the temple for a particular Gotipua dancer to perform on the boat before the deity. The boat is a float constructed on two boats with a red canopy over the dance-area.

Make-up and Costumes

Abhinay Chandrika, an important palm-leaf manuscript in Sanskrit text, but with an Oriya script commentary, written by Maheshwar Mahapatra in the 17th century, refers to the make-up and costumes required for Gotipua dancers. One of the manuscripts is in the possession of the present-day *guru* of Odissi dance, Kavichandra Shri Kalicharan Pattanaik, of Cuttack. The make-up indicated generally, is a buff colour base in powder-form which is applied on the face, collyrium is used to darken and elongate the eyes and eye-brows. A decorative pattern called *gorachana*, of a creeper like design, is painted on the forehead and encircles the eye-brows and runs down on to the cheeks. A beauty spot in the shape of a fly is placed on the chin. A *tika* or *tilak* mark on the forehead also adds beauty to the delicate face. Typical flower arrangement, specially devised for the hair-do, is called *pushpachuda* in the *Abhinaya Chandrika*. Two other types of flower arrangements are *ardha-baktaka* or semi-circular and *kati-beni* or a single plait hanging down the back.

A large number of ornaments were previously used by Gotipuas, as can be gathered from the several names mentioned in *Abhinaya Chandrika*. But nowadays the dancers use very few of them. *Chandra, alaka, ketaka,* are the names of some of those ornaments used for the head. For the ears, *kupa* are worn. Gotipuas also use several necklaces known by a variety of names such as *chapasari* and *padatilaka*. The arms are adorned with *tayita* and *karakankan* for the wrists. Around the waist are tied *bengapatia*—the silver belts.

For the costume, traditionally, the *pattasari* made of indigenous silk of bright colours, generally in some shades of red and nine yards in length, was worn. The *kanchula* or blouse, was also of a bright colour on which were sewn imitation stones. A length of cloth draped the hips and was tied in front, embellished with frills and was known as *nivibandh* and the cord called *jobha,* with *teasels* at both ends, was tied like a waist-band. Of late the *jobha* is not in vogue. This costume was similar to that used by the *maharis-devdasis*—the women temple dancers, in the past, the difference being in the manner of wearing the sari. The *pattasari* was worn tightly and it had an equal length of material on both sides which was caught up and tied in a knot near the navel.

Many changes in costume have been brought about now. The blouse is sometimes of shining glossy satin or velvet material. Instead of the traditional *pattasari*, a piece of bright coloured silk is used. There is however, some traditional order maintained. The Gotipua is still dressed as a girl. And finally, the anklets are tied on by the guru and the dancer is then ready for performance.

He is brought into the *akhada* and must first pay his obeisance to the Lord, after which he touches the feet of the guru. When the deity is brought in a palanquin procession to the *Chandan Pokhri*, the dancer is allowed to enter the boat, and, under the light of torches fixed in two stands in the boat, he dances before the sacred image. The guru plays the *pakhawaj* and a singer accompanies the dancer; the musicians occupy other boats. The theme is either from the Puranas or from *Gita Govinda*. Often during the *abalaya* or *abhinaya*—expressional dance—the dancer himself sings aş he dances. The dancing continues till the boat reaches the bank once again after the ceremonial boat-ride round the tank.

Often Gotipuas perform in the courtyards of certain temples.

For their services they receive some *dakshina* or offering. During *Jhoolan Yatra* for instance, Gotipuas dance at the *mukti mandap* or *jhoola mandap*.

Past Patronage

At first Gotipuas received patronage from the *akhada ghars* and the religious *mathas*. Certain zamindar families also maintained Gotipua parties for the entertainment of guests. The *akhadas* were established in several districts of Puri and Ganjam. It was in these districts that the *akhadas* flourished and patronage from local zamindars was forthcoming.

After Ramchandra Deva's rule, the next 300 years in Orissa was a period of turmoil for the State. Having lost its independence it was ruled in succession by the Pathans, Moghuls, Marathas and the British. These turbulent changes affected the religious, social and cultural life of the people. During the last century several other influences corrupted the dance of the Gotipuas, in particular the *Sakhi Nach* of the southern districts of Orissa. This dance belonged to the neighbouring Telugu regions. It was a voluptuous and sensuous dance of the *devdasis* and was imitated by the boys who performed the *Sakhi Nach*, which in turn influenced the Gotipua's dance, which lost much of its intrinsic beauty. To compete with touring *Jatra* theatrical companies and to please their patrons, an increasing vulgarity crept into the art of the Gotipuas. The latest danger of corruption is from the cinema and often the original Gotipua dance is completely disguised under a hotchpotch of so-called 'film' dancing.

What we see today is unfortunately, a form of dance that has come to us in a degenerate state. Indeed it is a poor imitation of Odissi dance. Luckily however, the present gurus of Odissi dance were Gotipuas trained during a period before decay had set in. Their efforts to save the dance, to reshape it and give it a new lease of life are very welcome. They are the torch-bearers of an unbroken tradition handed down in the traditional *guru-shishya parampara*. Foremost amongst them are the pupils of the late Guru Mohan Mahapatra—Shri Pankajcharan Das, Shri Debu Prasad Das and Shri Kelucharan Mahapatra, winner of the Sangeet Natak Akademi Award for Odissi dance.

18

KARAMA AND DALKHAI DANCE IN SAMBALPUR

Dhiren Pattanaik

Amongst the thirteen districts of Orissa, Sambalpur, is situated in the western-most part of the State which claims to possess a number of indigenous and colourful folk dances. The district consists of a wide expanse of fairly open country fringed by forest-clad hills on the west, north and east and intersected by the river Mahanadi. Half of the population are tribes and people of scheduled classes. They have a number of folk-dances closely associated with their social and religious life. Most of the dances deal with rituals and love and are danced by both men and women.

Karama Dance

Karama is the most colourful dance among the Binijhal, Kharia Oraon, Kisan and Kol tribes of the district. It is a ritual dance. It is performed in honour of "Karamasani" or 'Karamarani', the deity for granting children and who is also believed to be the cause of good and bad fortune. On the eleventh day of the full-moon of Bhadra the boys and girls go to the jungle singing and beating drums and cut a branch of the 'Karma' or 'Sal' tree, which is brought to a decorated circular place of the village where the dance takes place. The branch of the tree is ceremonially placed at the centre, where it is worshipped. The circular place is marked by the decoration of a long garland of mango leaves and water-lillies. After the installation of the branch, the village priest (locally known as

Jhankar) performs the rite by pouring liquor over it and making offerings of rice and sweet-meats. A fowl is also killed and the blood is offered to the branch. After the ritual is over the priest narrates the story of 'Karamasani', who is believed to have appeared to a man and promised that she would be present, whenever a branch of the 'Karam' or 'Sal' tree was broken. All the villagers give a patient hearing to the story and pay their obeissance to the deity, who is believed to be present there. Then they take country-liquor, prepared by them. Then songs are sung, drums are beaten and the young people dance vigorously.

In the beginning of the performance the dancers enter the dancing arena in two rows. The drummers (who play earthen drums, popularly known as Mandal), cymbal-players and singers accompany them with rhythmic steps. In first few rhythms they dance in different steps, individually, but maintain the symmetry. They then combine in twos and dance in sitting pose. The tempo slowly rises and all of them sit face to face and stretch their legs. Then they bend towards the front and the sides keeping rhythm in ankle-bells. Lastly, they get up and dance in pairs in a quicker tempo by placing each other's left hands on the shoulders. The dance has a rich repertory. Every change is marked by a cut in music with movemetns of the wriggling of the body. This dance of Binijhal dancers is one of the light-hearted freshness combined with a youthful energy which makes it a most charming and enjoyable spectacle.

During the performance, the dancers do not sing, but shout *Hai, Hai* according to the rhythm of the drums. The costume of the dance is extremely beautiful and rich in colour. The dancers, drummers and singers wear a turban of red cloth and beautifully designed peacock feathers as head dress; a red shirt of local design and a scanty coloured cloth (which hangs up to the knees) as garment, skilfully designed armlets, bangles and girdles made out of small conch-shells and a long garland of ankle bells to mark the time beats. Peculiarly, each of the dancers hold a mirror in the right or left hand while they dance. It is perhaps to see and appreciate their colourful costume, which is mainly to attract the young girls, who watch patiently and talk to each other about the dancers, particularly those whom they appreciate. This is because special facilities are given to young girls on festival days to mix with the other sex and they are allowed to make their own selection for marriage. But they are extremely strict regarding any liaison between them and men of higher castes.

After the dance of the males, the young girls enter the arena. The former group disperse and watch the performance of the girls. The dance of the girls is different from the former. They hold hands in different ways in different dances, sometimes they simply hold hands, sometimes hands are placed on the neighbours' waistband or are crossed, front or back; sometimes they are placed on the neighbours' shoulders and sometimes they dance arm in arm. When hands are simply held, they are swung backwards and forwards, energetically, in rhythm with the fast or slow tempo of the dance. When they get very close together, arms are raised up from elbow. Bending the body forward and backwards, right and left, bending the knees, dancing in half sitting position, crossing the hands of each other and clapping, are some of the peculiar characteristics of this dance. The girls always move in lines in a semi-circular pattern and complete circles while dancing in the wide circular place. While dancing they sing different tunes—a long song praying for rain is a special feature of the festival. This indicates the tradition of nature-worship of the primitive people. Peculiarly, the girls do not wear any special costume for the occasion as the boys.

Towards the end of the dance the boys join the girls and they dance in separate lines. At this moment the dance reaches a faster tempo. The dance continues till the morning, after which the branch is taken away in procession and thrown into a village tank or the nearest stream. This practice is prevalent among all the tribes. This is the style of the dance of Binijhals, who are the Kshatriyas or the ruling class among the tribes and are said to be the earliest inhabitants of the district.

After the Karama dance is over, the Binijhals have a festival called the 'Sua' dance. Young girls go about from village to village singing and dancing accompanied by drummers and Gond musicians. They are entertained in each village they visit and are lodged comfortably for the night. Next morning they dance for five or six hours and then proceed to another village, dancing, singing and beating drums. Love is the main theme of the songs. Due to the influence of modern civilisation this practice is slowly dying out.

The technique of the Karama dance varies a little from tribe to tribe. The Khariyas, Kisans and Oraons dance in a circular pattern, where men and women dance together. It is always headed by a leader, generally a man at the head of the line. Only the best of dancers becomes his neighbour. Very young girls and children join the tail-end to learn the steps. When the dancing grows fast, the dancers at the tail-end drop out to let the experienced dancers show their skill. The dancers hold hands in different ways in different dances, sometimes they simply hold hands and sometimes hands are placed on the neighbours' waist-band or are crossed. It is the legs and the feet which play the principal part in the dance. The dance begins lightly with simple steps forward and backward, left and right then gradually the steps grow smaller and faster, growing more and more complicated, until the dance reaches its height, then it goes gradually back to the first steps as the music leads to give the dancers rest. The dancers have no special costume for the occasion.

Karama is also known as 'Keli Kadam' festival among some tribes. This particular dance-form is also performed during Dushera, Phagunpuni, Bhai Jauntia and some other festive occasions. This dance is also prevalent in Mayurbhanj, Sundergarh, Bolangir and Dhenkanal districts of Orissa. Rituals being the same, the technique of the dance and music differ from the abovementioned tribes.

Dalkhai Dance

This form of dance is performed by the young girls of Binijhal, Saura, Kuda-Nirdha and some other tribes of the district. Sometimes young girls of scheduled class also take part. Dushera, Bhai Jauntia, Phagunpuni and other festive days are the occasions for this dance.

In the beginning of the performance the young girls stand in a line or in a semi-circular pattern and sing songs, which are commonly known as Dalkhai songs. They sing for a while and then dance by bending forward to a half-sitting position. While singing they do not dance and the *Dhol* remains the only accompanying drum. During the dance different varieties of drums and wind-instruments are played. These are *Dhol*, a big drum which is played with one stick in the left hand and the right side is played by the bare hand; *Nisan*, a one-sided drum usually two feet in diameter and made of iron case, is played by two sticks by both the hands; *Tamki*, a tiny onesided drum of six inches in diameter, is played with two sticks, *Tasa*, (a kind of drum) and *Mahuri* (wind-instrument). All these instruments form a rich orchestra of folk-music, which is inspiring and vigorous in rhythm and varies according to the various movements of the dance. The Dhol-player dances with the girls and other musicians sit by the side of the dancing place and play. Most of the musicians are from 'untouchable' class.

This particular dance of the girls is of explosive vitality. Different movements of the hands, legs, knees and hips which are characteristics of this dance are given primary importance.

The dance has no special costume for the girls. But during the dance they place a piece of cloth on the shoulders and hold the two ends in both the hands separately. While dancing they move their hands forward and backward alternatively.

19

THE MAHARI

Sadashiva Ratha Sharma

Devadasi dance in the temple of Lord Jagannath at Puri is also known as the *Mahari* dance. The devadasis are called Maharis which literally means, according to some, one who is deeply in love with Lord. Dancing has remained a very important and indispensable item in the daily rituals (*seva*) of Lord Jagannath since the time of Ganga rulers of Utkal in the 12th century. Besides the inscriptions of the Ganga rulers there are also some old treatises and literatures which hold the proof for the oldness of this ritual in the temple of Lord Jagannath.

We also find dancing as a ritual in the temple of Lord Jagannath, mentioned in Agni Purana, Vishnu Purana, Srimad Bhagavat, Padma Purana and Skanda Purana.

Chodaganga Dev who ruled Utkal in the twelfth century is credited to have first introduced devadasi dancing in the temple of Lord Jagannath. He established seven streets (*sahis*) for the servants (*sebayat*) of the Lord and one of these streets known by the name Anga Alasa Patana was intended for the Maharis alone. Chodaganga Dev introduced several ceremonies (Jatra) of the Lord Jagannath in a year. It is of interest to note that dancing and singing are associated with almost all these ceremonies.

The 'Maharis' in olden days, enjoyed a place of esteem in the society. Girls of respectable families took it as an honourable profession. The Maharis were of six categories : Bhitar Gauni, Bahar Gauni, Nachuni, Patauri, Raj Angila and Gahan Mahari.

Improvements were made in Devadasi or Mahari dancing during the 16th century. Prataprudra Dev was a great patron of dance and music. He introduced one more item, Ekanta Seva or Palanka Pakhari Seva in the daily services of the Maharis. Ramananda Pattnaik, a great Vaishnava and poet of the time used to dress up the Maharis himself and teach them the arts of Abhinaya and the techniques of Nritta.

Later, two officers named Mina Nahak and Sahi Nahak were posted in each street to regulate the services of the Maharis. These officers were supposed to see that the Maharis had a chaste and honourable life and remain dutiful in their services. I am quoting below an extract of a royal order which I found in the possession of an old Mahari named Buli.

"The order prohibits the Maharis from having physical contact with men. They should not dance in any festival except those of Lord Jagannath. After initiation in Vaishnavism they should adorn their body with marks of Tilak and Kali and should take Tulshi Kanthi. They should not take food cooked at home nor should they speak to any male on the days they are to dance before the Lord. They should wear clean clothes. They should be led to the temple by the Mina Nahak on the occasion of the performance. While dancing they should not look at the pilgrim audience. They should dance according to the directions in the Shastra and think of themselves as servants of the Lord. They should not touch any Sudra. The dancer and the singer should progress in perfect cooperation. There should not be any flaw in Tal and Swara. They should dance in the following Tals : Pahapata, Sariman, Parameshwar Malasree, Harachandi Malashri, Chandana Jhula, Srimangala Bachanika, Jhuti Ath Tali and should make Abhinaya of the songs from Gita Govinda."

I heard many old Maharis quoting names of several *shastras* such as 'Devadasi Nrutya Paddhati' of Narayan Mishra, 'Nachuni Bidhi' of Madhu Patanaik, 'Niladri Nacha' of Mukta Mahari. Unfortunately, none of those MSS have come to me as yet.

The Mahari comes to the Garuda Stambha in the temple being accompanied by the Raj Guru who holds a gold mounted cane in his hand as a sign of authority. The dance is performed under his supervision. The Mahari begins her dance after saluting the Lord and Raj Guru.

In dance, the Maharis follow certain accepted movements of the legs. These movements are named according to the placement of the legs. These are called *Bhumi* or ground, which are mainly of five kinds—Chauka, Minadandi, Bartula, Ghera and Dwimukha.

Chauka means a square—the area within which the dancer completes her performance. The dancer beginning her first item from the centre of the ground proceeds, while dancing towards the corner of the place and with turns at each corner she rounds an imaginary square sized area. After this she turns to her place of starting.

Minadandi movement resembles the diagram of a skeleton of a fish. The dancer moves forward from the centre stretching the fore parts of the legs at two sides at each foot step. On reaching the end of the ground, she turns back and repeats the movement, backwards. Her feet move always in the figure of a skeleton of a fish.

The dancer, at times, comes forward and revolving round herself at certain intervals encircles the imaginary ground and comes to the centre from the back. This movement is known by the name of *Bartula* or a circle.

The rapid encircling around the centre by the Mahari is known as *Ghera*.

The stretching of feet in their natural position towards their respective sides is called *Dwimukha*, that is, double faced.

The Maharis speak of six types of Chari or Chali now popularly accepted in Orissi dancing : Goithi, Chapuani, Kada Ghosara, Thia Puchi, and Phuhania.

Walking with the support of the heels is known as Goithi Chali. The beginning of the dance on the fore parts of the feet with the heels raised is known as Chapuani. Moving with a foot stretched sideways one after another is known as Kada Ghosara.

The left foot should be stretched in the left and the right foot on the right. Moving forward resting the body in a sitting position on fore parts of the feet with the heels raised is known as Thia Puchi. The lifting of one foot a bit upward in the side by keeping it by the side of the other foot and repeating the same action with the other foot is known as Puhania Chali.

It is really a misfortune that true techniques of Orissi dance amongst the Maharis have now come to total eclipse. They do not consider their profession honourable. They have just preserved the tradition without having any devotion or sincerity for it. There are at present only two or three old Maharis who could tell something about the techniques of Orissi dance. The facts I have gathered from them have been stated above. It requires further survey and research to establish as to how much of it is fact and how much fiction.

20

CHHAU NACHA

A. Chowdhury

Chhau dance is prevalent in Mayurbhanj in Orissa, Sareikela in Bihar and Purulia in West Bengal. Under the royal patronage of the different princely states in this area, Chhau was nurtured and developed. In the course of stylisation of the costumes and the use of masks it branched off into three different schools. In Purulia and Sareikela masks are used but in Mayurbhanj there is no mask. Here we would be discussing the Sareikela and Mayurbhanj forms of Chhau dance.

In Sareikela and Mayurbhunj, there are a large variety of tribes belonging to Austric and Munda groups. These tribes are shift cultivators or food-gatherers. Though Chhau dance is an expression of village culture it has many purely tribal elements in it. The people who perform these dances almost invariably belong to the scheduled or backward classes like *Nats*, *Bhands*, *Bhumiyas*, *Paiks* and others. Mayurbhanj Chhau is performed by the priests amongst the scheduled caste. Chhau dance gives an insight into the inter-action between the different levels of Indian society. Co-existence of many layers of civilisation and culture and multiplicity of meaning and symbolism is evident in this dance-form. Here we have a dance-form where the tribal, village and urban culture, the *Margi*, the *Desi*, the *Natyadharmi* and the *Lokadharmi* are blended together to make a new whole.

It is said that the word *Chhau* is derived from the Sanskrit word *chhaya* which means shadow or image. This appears to be farfetched. In Oriya, Chhau means to hunt or to attack stealthily.

The word Chhau has three colloquial Oriya derivatives :
chhauri (armour), *chhauni* (military camp) and *chhauka* (quality
of attacking stealthily). It is said that Chhau dance originated
from the martial dance *Pharikhanda Khela* (playing with the
sword and the shield). But Chhau dance is basically a ritual
dance. Gradually, it grew to classical heights with elaborate
stylisation and developed a sophisticated grammar of movements, tala etc.

During the reign of Maharaj Krishna Chandra Bhanj Deo
of Mayurbhanj Chhau came into prominence. The *bhangis* and
bhavas of Chhau were further developed by his son Sri Ramchandra Bhanj Deo. The sophisticated theory of the intricate
pattern of movements of this dance form was further developed
during the reign of Sri Pratap Chandra Bhanj Deo.

Chhau dances are generally performed during the Chaitra
Parva and is held on the *Chaitra Samkranti* corresponding
roughly to April 13. Thirteen days before the Samkranti a
series of rituals begin. Thirteen devotees called *bhakta* or
bhagata drawn from different castes that are considered lower,
perform some religious rituals daily. They wear deep red dhotis
and like the Brahmin wear the sacred thread. They fast, take
ritual bath, visit the temple of Goddess Ambika and then proceed to offer worship to lord Shiva, at a consecrated place.
They perform the fire-walking ritual called *Nian Pata*. The
Bhaktas also perform a ritual where the devotee is suspended by
their feet on a pole over a flaming fire. This is called *Jhula
Pata*. They sometimes walk on thorns. These and other ceremonies are performed on the 26th day of the month of Chaitra
when a pitcher of water is brought out to herald the beginning
of the festival.

The dance begins with *Rangabaja*. This is performed behind the screen. It is essentially a musical invocation. This
is followed by the instrumentalists playing a tune with which
the different characters appear on the stage. This is known as
Chali (walking). The characters appear in their different
dharanas (stances). After the characters appear on the stage
his *nacha* begins. Here the theme is introduced but very little
dramatic action takes place. *Natki* is the final phase performed
to an accelerated tempo, where the dramatic action is heigh-

tened. The dance is presented to the accompaniment of *dhol* (a drum played with the palm and fingers of the left hand and a blunt stick in the right); *nagara* (a hemispherical drum played with two thin sticks); *chadihadi* (cylindrical drum played with stick); *dhamsa* (bowl shaped kettle drum) and *mahoori* (indigenous wind instrument very much like *shehnai*). The tunes played by these instruments have much in common with folk and Orissi songs.

The basic steps and gaits from which the dance develops are called *topkas* and *uflis*, performed formally with a sword in the right and shield in the left hand. These are modified forms of exercises which in ancient times were performed by the soldiers to tune up their bodies to play the hand-held weapons with the agility of lightning.

Topka may be defined as the style of gait in which the imagery is conjured through the flexions of the body and the footwork follows perfectly. In *uflis* the legs convey the imagery and the body moves in agreement.

Uflis and *topkas* interwoven purposefully becomes a *bhangi* or a dance unit. *Bhangis* properly syntaxed delineate the theme of the dance, build up drama and give meaning to the rhythmic movements. There is no *hasta-mudra* in Chhau. This is because in the formative stage the movement of hand was restricted by holding of some weapon. All the units of the movement are classified from the point of view of the nature of the movement, strong, quick, terse cutting and fluid, liquid and elastic. They are known as *Hathiyardhara* (holding of the weapon); *Kalikata* (to cut with a weapon) and *Kalibhanga* (bending of the softest twig). *Hathiyardhara* and *Kalikata* suggests *Tandava* movements and *Kalibhanga*, *Lasya* movements.

The most important units of movements are the six *chalis* (the gaits), six *topkas*, thirty-six *uflis* and 250 *up-uflis*. The *uflis* incorporate movements relating to agricultural operations, daily routine of the housewife, toilet preparations, war-drills and gaits of different animals. Some others depict the working of the human mind and play of certain emotions. Mayurbhanj Chhau emphasises the movements of flying *gandharva* of Natyashastra suggesting the elevation of the lower limb and is unique in terms of classical dance movements.

Myths and legends of Hinduism are depicted in the group dance-dramas such as *Tamadic Krishna*, *Garud Vahana*, *Samudramanthana*, *Ahalya Udhara* etc.

The royal family of Sareikela was the patron and performers of Chhau. Rajkumar Suddendra, the prince of Sareikela is the best exponent of this tradition. The dance is performed annually at the *Chaitra Parva* festival. The festival has elaborate rituals in honour of Kali and celebrates the glory of Shiva. In this form of dance, the dancer wears a mask and keeps mute. Only instrumental music accompanies the dance.

The Chhau mask is made of dark clay. The nose and the eyes are fashioned by a sharp steel instrument (*Karni*). After the mould becomes dry, the clay is scooped out from the hollow of the mask by the *Karni* and the mask is scrubbed, polished and painted.

The themes are *Dheebar* (fishermen), *Astradanda* (swordplay) and *Sabara* (hunter). The dance is either solo or duet; never a group dance as in Mayurbhanj form of Chhau. There are sophisticated and difficult movements, inner tension, vivid body-expression in *Nabik* (boatman), *Mayura* (peacock), *Banaviddha* (the arrow-stricken deer), *Nabik* describes a man and a woman in a storm-tossed boat. The woman clings to the man for security. This gives the man strength and he fights the storm. Sudden misery brings them together and they emerge triumphant.

There are nine types of *topkas* and 23 types of *uflis* in Sareikela Chhau. The use of mask here necessitated a different type of stylisation in which the movements have to be more symbolic. This is a highly stylised form of dance. The interpretation of most themes is metaphysical. The rhythms occasionally have difficult patterns. The most commonly used *ragas* are *Desh* and *Malkauns*. Sareikela Chhau is either a duet or a solo dance. Sareikela masks are symbolic rather than descriptive, of the characters played. The mask not only stands at the focal point of the dance but also conditions the formation of *bhangis*. The *angikabhinaya* (expression through body movements) of Sareikela Chhau is so unique, so expressive that even without *vachikabhinaya* (expression through songs, words), and *mukhabhinaya* (expression through facial movements) the communication of *bhava* is complete and aesthetically most satisfying. Sareikela Chhau is poetic, projecting life and beauty in rhythms and in harmonious movements of the body.

Chhau dance as a distinctive form—free, fluent, dynamic and intense; is a fusion of tribal, folk and classical styles.

21

SAHI YATRA

Durgadas Mukhopadhyay

Sahi Yatra, a unique form of folk-theatre from Orissa, is performed in the bylanes of Puri. *Sahi* means 'alley' or 'back-street', *Yatra* refers to movement or procession. *Sahi Yatra* is an enactment of life through the streets—life that is moving, flamboyant, vigorous and unending. The Yatra starts to the tune of musical instruments, the procession moves and people grow restless, involved, tired as they concentrate on singing, dancing, gesturing to the accompaniment of dramatic drumming and the enactment of sequences that are very much part of their own lives.

During the first month of spring, Sahi Yatra is performed continuously for three days. Whether rich or poor, of high or low caste, everyone is either actor, singer, instrumentalist or part of the audience. Through the narrow lanes of the city and at the very centre of this organised procession the main character : the *Naga-Saja* (who represents a particular manifestation of Lord Jagannath), moves slowly, languorously, sometimes violently. He wears a papier-mache crown decorated with paddystalk. He has a long upturned moustache and a thick black beard. A tiger-skin is wound around his chest and he wears anklets of bark. His waist supports a bow-shaped tail of twenty ornaments. He moves rhythmically, often vigorously. When he grows tired he is quietly replaced and the procession moves on.

Sahi Yatra is an integral processional theatre. It depicts joy, sorrows, agonies and ecstacy, inconsistencies, double-standards, elements of protest in a social system.   Humour and satire is the starting point of this processional theatre.   The *Patuar* (life through procession) is a conglomeration of crystalised, stylised prototypes of society who are exposed, analysed and ridiculed.   The procession is colourful and comic to the core. We see characters like *Kela-Kelini*, *Shabara-Shabri*, *Burda-Burhi*. *Kela-Kelini* are two big (12-15 feet) decorated masked unusual human figures.   The inside is hollow and actors get inside this huge structure and manipulate the movement of these husband and wife comic figures. The figures are mobile and unusual with a big head, long nose, huge bulging tummy and long decorated legs. They sing comic songs which ridicule the inconsistencies in social life.   The stories deal with businessman and his wife, the king and his concubines and sycophants, the pundits etc. *Shabara-Shabari* are tribal husband and wife to evoke curiosity in a different life pattern.   They are comical and satirise situations and episodes from life around.   These characters, though stylised depict real-life situations through humour and satire and are irresistible to the children in the crowd.   The blending of surprise, satire and irony as well as a touch of realism in it is superb.

There is stylised bull-fighting as a part of the procession. These are big, hollow figures of bull, inside which a person manipulates the movement and gestures like the charging of the bulls. The most interesting is the red lips of the bull sprouting out, moving in different directions, manipulated by a string by the unseen person inside the bull. The bull-fight is powerful, ferocious and fascinating. It provides entertainment to the children and the adult alike.   There is also the real fight of well-fed, ferocious rams.   These rams belong to different *jagas* or *akharas*. They are properly fed and looked after throughout the year.   The prestige of a locality depends on the result of this ram fight.   It can be compared with the cock-fighting and pigeon-flying of Lucknow. Children wear masks and paint their bodies as tigers, leopards or lions. They move in rhythmic gestures and the fight between the tiger and leopard is presented with artistic sophistry. There is fierce sword-fighting and fighting with *lathis* as part of the procession.

In this long procession, musicians, drummers and singers

are in the front; then comes the *patuar*, then the enactment of subplots through gestures accompanied by little singing and vigorous drumming.

Sahi Yatra is normally performed in the first month of spring. But it may also be performed during the different *beshas* (festivals) of Lord Jagannath depending on the preparation of the *jagas* or *akharas*. There are 19 such *beshas* in a year.

Several inter-related plays are enacted around the *Naga-Saja*. The theme and content of these plays are normally borrowed from the Puranas, Ramayana and Mahabharata and also from local folk-tales and folk-songs. The stories of *Vritryasura, Daityasura, Hiranyakasipu* and *Kaliya Daman* for instance derive from the Puranas, yet as the procession makes its way through the streets folk myths spontaneously weave in and out of these events.

There is no authentic history of the growth and development of *Sahi Yatra*. *Anarghyaraghava*, a Sanskrit play written by Murari Misra in 850 A.D. provides possibly the first reference to *Sahi Yatra*.

Lavanod bela banani tamala taru
Kandarasya tribhuvan mouli mandanam mohanilmonou
Kamala kuchakalas keli kasturika potrankurasya
Bhagwatah purushottamasya *sahiyatrayam*
Upsthaniya sabhasadah.

"On the sea-shore, amidst the tamala trees in the forest of the blue mountain—the crown of the three worlds; Lord Krishna is smeared with the musk decorations on the pitcher-like breasts of Radha. Oh, the connoisseurs! please join in the *Sahi Yatra* of Lord Krishna".

The Puri Temple is said to have been rebuilt in 1190-1198 by Ananga Bhima Deva, and earlier the Shabars and Nishads (hunters and food-gathering tribals) had been accepted as *Dayitapati* or attendants of the temple of Lord Jagannath (as early as the reign of King Indradumnya). However, with the Brahmin supremacy of the Muktimandap by the time of king Yayati Kesari these Shabars were denied entry to the temple altogether. It is possible that ostracised from religious society in this way, the natural vitality of tribal feeling found expression in the *Veera-rasa* and *Bhayanaka-rasa* that continue with devotional attitude towards Lord Jagannath as a close family member, a friend, benefactor, saviour and destroyer of evils (in the form of demons who devour the universal principle of Right).

The renowned Oriya writer, Surendra Mohanty says that to trace the origin in time of *Sahi Yatra* is futile in terms of the available measurements of time in our everyday life.

The particular character of Naga-Saja is associated with the *Nagarjunabesha* aspect of Lord Jagannath. The sub-plots revolve around the *Naga-Saja* and are sung to the accompaniment of the *dholak, changu, ghunti, ghanta* and *nagara* together with the *muhri (*or *kahari manjira).* The stories are known to the audience. Any member of the audience may spontaneously participate in the singing, the dancing or the acting itself, afterwards reverting to the role of audience. The spontaneity is what makes *Sahi Yatra* unique. The songs in Oriya are Puranic with a local flavour.

> *Artryatranar parandhana mote chhadi chali galure*
> *Hey kalakalia-kainchmalia mo jiba pasari delure*
> *Tote chhadi muin haribi parana chitkar chhadibi muin re*
> *Girikandara mo shakarkanda lova tu pasari delure*

"Oh the beloved of the oppressed, you deserted me. Oh Krishna, who wears bead-necklace, you made me forget my life. I would die without you, cry I must : I am like the sweet potato, you made me forget my greed."

> *Hanibi, katibi, jalibi, chalibi tora a maya sansarare*
> *Marile maribi na bhuli paribi to maharanka paranare*

"Charge, kill, put fire, proceed in this world of illusion. You would die but would never be able to forget this life of immense attachment."

The form of Sahi Yatra is basically that of a musical play with its structure founded in *tala*. Starting at one end of a particular street and moving through a series of galis it will end at the same place in the same street from which it started. There are several *akharas* or *jagas* or troupes of Sahi Yatra and there is fierce rivalry among them.

The main character of the play is magnanimous, larger-than-life presence who is surrounded by smaller figures and who is the representation and fusion of the sorrows, struggle, happiness, resistance and ultimate victory of human life. In this, Sahi Yatra moves beyond the limitations of time, space and environment; here everything is moving forward towards a strongly sensed destination. The inherent meaning of this form is very old, based as it is on several life times' observation, identification and faith in life's meaning. This form is decaying. One reason for this may be that the modern urban values can no longer support such a metaphysic. Competition from mass media and lack of patronage may also explain its decay. Recent technical and verbal vulgarisation can only be understood in terms of present socio-economic pressures.

However, this particular form is definitely potent and deserves further exploration.

22

NAUTANKI

Ashok Chakradhar

The Hindi-speaking North Indian villages are connoisseurs of *Nautanki*. It is their own folk-theatre. News that a particular Nautanki troupe is going to perform in a certain village spreads like wildfire. Thousands of people come to the tent lured by the call of *nakara* or drum. It could be *Sultana Daku*, *Amar Singh Rathod* or *Satya Harishchander* or any other popular Nautanki play, the audience is familiar with the story, songs and even the dialogues of the play. They might have seen the same Nautanki play a couple of times before. They sit through the performance from evening to dawn, engrossed in the rhythm of the powerful *nakara* and the deep throated voice of the singers.

The origin of this form of folk-theatre and the history of its development is controversial, but Hathras and Kanpur are considered to be its main centres. These two schools of Nautanki are similar in structure—only the presentations differ. In Hathras the stress is on the lyrics and the style of singing whereas in Kanpur the emphasis is on dialogue and the style of acting. There are hundreds of troupes in both these areas but out of the famous troupes mention can be made of *Brij Lok Manch* of Hathras and *Sri Krishna Pahalwan's* troupe of Kanpur. The other important *Akharas* or schools of Nautanki are Saharanpur, Muzaffarnagar and Kanauj, each named after the town in which it originated. Some theatrical forms closely resembling Nautanki are the *Bhagat* of Agra, the *Sang* of

Haryana, the *Khyal* of Rajasthan and *Manch* of Madhya Pradesh.

It is difficult to trace the history of the moving folk tradition particularly of the folk-theatre forms. Nautanki has been changing its structure continuously over centuries modifying itself to the needs of changing situations. The first mention of Nautanki is found in *Ain-e-Akbari*—a 15th century treatise. Reference is made to a group of mendicants who used to preach during the night imitating and enacting the religious leaders of the time. Later these men formed their own troupe and travelled all over North India. Some scholars are of the opinion that Nautanki started as a form of lyric singing in Punjab in the 12th century and later these troupes moved eastward. But it is strange that one does not find Punjabi words in any style of Nautanki; its vocabulary being pure Hindustani.

An important 19th century musical drama was *Indrasabha* (The court of God Indra) by Agha Hassan Amanat, the famous Urdu poet of Lucknow. Amanat used traditional melodies, folk tunes and seasonal dances along with his dramatic lyrics. The operatic play went into many editions during his lifetime. Various Nautanki troupes modified its characters, situations, and melodies. Its popularity inspired Nautanki writers who sought to emulate its whimsical and other worldly atmosphere of fairies, devils, gods, princes, wizards and dancers.

There are different opinions about the name *Nautanki* itself. Some believe that Nautanki is derived from the Sanskrit word *Natak* or drama. The story from which Nautanki takes its name, tells of the Princess Nautanki of Multan (Rani Nautanki). She was exceptionally beautiful. In a neighbouring state lived two brothers Bhup Singh and Phool Singh. One day the younger brother Phool Singh—handsome and adventurous, returns from the hunt and asks his sister-in-law to serve him food quickly. She taunts him saying that he is behaving as if he were the husband of the beautiful princess Nautanki. Phool Singh, insulted and hurt, leaves home, vowing that he will not return until he has married Nautanki. His faithful friend Yashwant Singh accompanies him. On reaching Multan they meet the flower-woman of the palace and beg her to allow them to stay in her hut. Everyday this flower-woman carries a garland of fresh flowers to the princess. Phool Singh, expert in the art of floral decorations offers to weave a garland for the princess if his hostess will cook for him. The flower woman takes the garland to the princess who suspects that someone else has prepared it. The flower-woman explains that her nephew's young wife has been on a short visit and that she has prepared the garland. The princess commands her to produce the young woman before her and the flower-woman returns to her hut greatly perturbed. Phool Singh calms her by suggesting that he is superb in the art of disguise and would not be recognised if he wears women's clothes. The flower-woman takes Phool Singh disguised as a beautiful woman to the princess who is struck by 'her' beauty. She offers her friendship and insists that Phool Singh stay in her chamber. He agrees. At night the princess sighs that if Phool Singh were a man she would marry him. Phool Singh asks her to close her eyes, meditate on the household deity and invoke the deity's blessings to turn one of them into a man. This the princess does and when she opens her eyes she finds that her companion has been turned into a handsome companion. A love scene follows. In the morning the palace-maid reports the matter to the king who orders the young man to be arrested and killed. Nautanki, carrying a sword and a cup of poison reaches the spot where Phool Singh is awaiting death. She drives off the executioners and challenges her father. The king deeply moved, agrees to her marriage with Phool Singh. Phool Singh returns home with his bride.

Almost every composer of Nautanki has mentioned this episode. Even though there might not be any princess named Nautanki in history, the impression of this episode is so strong in the minds of the people of North India that the romance has stayed.

Nautanki is similar in style to *Bhagat* but there are some differences between these two forms. As is evident from the name, *Bhagat* has religious associations. Nautanki is a commercialised, secularised form of Bhagat whereas the themes, lyrics and the stage itself are the same. Each guru or teacher of Bhagat has his own *akhara* or pit. There is friendly

competition among the different pits. The guru of the pit is
the writer, director and composer. After lighting the sacred
lamp in praise of Ganesh, (in which the actor Ganesh himself
dances on the stage) the actual performance starts. The same
ritual is to be found in Nautanki but it does not carry the same
importance. The religious sentiment soon fades and immedi-
ately after the ritual, performance starts straight away with the
dance by the girls. Then the actual story is enacted.

Gradually *Nautanki* started becoming troupe-based rather
than pit-based. Nautanki is a vocation for all its performers. The pits of Bhagat would receive donations and contributions from the richer section of society and these patrons
would maintain the prestige of a particular pit.

After the munity of 1857, the colonials realised the impact
of Bhagat's performers on the masses, and proceeded to exploit
these practitioners' art for furthering their own cause. To
divert the attention of the masses from revolutionary sentiments
the gurus were forced to write vulgar, erotic and titillating
Bhagats. It is said that Bhagwati Prasad of the Kalangi
troupe was offered ten thousand rupees to write a lovestory
named *Sabzpari*. Bhagat was gradually getting commercialised.
Except for few pits in Agra, Bhagat is almost extinct. Mean-
while, Nautanki started becoming popular with the decline of
Bhagat tradition.

Nautanki is a musical play in which prose-dialogue and
dances are also used. The music of Nautanki is not classical in
nature though based on the classical *ragas*. *Nagara* is the main
musical instrument in Nautanki Other instruments used are
—the *Sarangi*, Harmonium and *Dholak*. *Doha choubola*, *Kada
Daur Chatti* are the metres normally used in recitation. After
one or two lines the *nagara* is played for the same duration.
The tempo of the narration is rather slow. The reputation of
a particular troupe depends on the range of the singer and it is
true that it is difficult to compete with them in their colaratura
singing. As far as the language of Nautanki is concerned
there is no single dialect but a mixture of the different dialects
of North India. As compared to the *Hathras* school, relatively
more Urdu is used in the Nautankis of Kanpur.

There are thousands of Nautanki plays. The Nautankis of

Braja are mainly written by Inderman and his disciple Nathuram Gaud. Srikrishna Pahalwan has written many Nautankis for the *Kanpur* school. These writers have their own troupe, they themselves are the singers. They have written Nautankis on different themes based on stories from the Ramayana, Mahabharata and Puranas, folk-stories etc. The main *rasa* or essence of emotions depicted are *Sringara rasa* or love; and *Vira rasa* on bravery.

Nautanki writers have adapted locally popular love stories for their plays. *Laila-Majnu* and *Siya Posh* are some such Nautankis. There are also Nautankis like *Amar Singh Radhod* based on historical themes. Some Nautankis are based on true stories of bravery such as *Sultana Daku* and *Andhi Dulhan*. Srikrishna Pahalwan has written Nautankis based on social themes like *Beti ka Sauda* (Sale of the Daughter) *Garib Kisan* (The Poor Peasant) and *Bharat Durdasa* (Decay of India). Nautanki writers never had to face the problem of 'the unity of three'. Their imagination crossed the barriers of time, space and environment. Sita in their plays could dance like a prostitute. The dialogues may be filled with exaggeration and melodrama. Yet all these taken together, created a new dramatic consciousness. The more it was influenced by Parsi Theatre the more urban vulgarity and obscenity started creeping into the performances. The Kanpur troupe became a hunting ground of prostitutes. Use of obscene and vulgar songs based on film-tunes started increasing. As compared to the Kanpur troupe, the Braja group was less vulgarised. The director of *Braj Lok Manch* of Hathras, Radheshyam made significant contribution to direction by maintaining the purity of Nautanki and restraining its tendency towards vulgarity.

At present, urban theatre with its limitations and deadend future is attempting new grounds in folk-tradition. Plays are being produced where Nautanki form and style is being used. One can mention *Bakri* written by Sarveshwar Dayal Saxena and *Ek Satya Harishchandra* of Lakshmi Narayan Lal. Urban audiences seem to have appreciated these productions. But the question remains how meaningful and proper is it to make these folk-art forms a show-piece or museum-piece in the name of modification and modernisation. New Nautankis must be

written, but it must be kept in mind that these are not meant
for urban audiences alone.   Nautanki is basically folk-theatre
and it can best come into its own with a strong rural support.
The diluted adaptation and presentation of Nautanki in cities
can be appreciated for its novelty but it is definitely unfair to
the rich folk-tradition.

23

SHADOW THEATRE OF INDIA
Jiwan Pani

Shadow theatre is different to all other forms of theatre including puppet theatre. Limited of necessity to a highly stylised convention the shadow theatre has proved itself an artistic medium of rare and delicate charm. Shadows present objects in an unknown dimension. Bertolt Brecht believed that from the artist's perspective every so-called ordinary object should appear strange. Shadow play creates that type of strangeness. A real world of space is created on stage in which flat figures, usually made of leather, are lightly pressed on a translucent screen with a strong source of light behind them. The audience sits on the other side of the screen where it can see the shadows move as the figures are manipulated. Thus spectators and actors separated by the light screen are placed as if in different spaces. The spectator's feeling of isolation is heightened by the surrounding darkness. He does not directly experience the figures or the play, he only sees the image, the projection. The light screen which filters and modifies the action, isolates the puppeteers who presents a projection of his thoughts for the spectator to interpret and reassemble into a new image. It is not the puppet figure in his hand but the image on the screen that decides his mode of manipulation. He translates them into a moving picture in shadow. In the mind of the audience these moving shadow-compositions are re-translated into happenings. This is what gives shadow theatre its subtle excitement.

It is usually regarded as an ancient form of theatre and some scholars trace its origin to China where there is still a potent shadow tradition in which ancestor-worship and magic play their part. Other scholars are of opinion that shadow theatre originated in India since there are references to the various forms of puppetry in the literary works of early centuries B.C. From these references it appears that about 2000 years ago shadow theatre along with other forms of puppetry flourished in India as a very intimate part of our group life particularly in the villages.

Under the impact of industrialisation and especially since the move towards popular cinema has claimed mass attention in both the urban and rural regions, the folk and traditional performing arts of India have begun to languish in remote corners without either connoisseurship or patronage.

Fortunately, the tradition of shadow theatre survives in Orissa, Kerala, Andhra Pradesh and Karnataka. While the shadow puppets of Orissa and Kerala project silhouette-like shadow, in black, the Andhra and Karnataka puppets throw coloured shadows on the screen.

The Orissa shadow theatre locally known as *Ravanchchaya* presents the Rama legend and follows the text of *Vichitra Ramayana* by Vishwanath Khutia, a medieval Oriya poet. The puppets are made of deer-skin and are conceived in bold dramatic poses. Many props such as trees, mountains, chariots, etc. are also used for creating appropriate illusions. Although, *Ravanchhaya* puppets are smller in size (the largest not more than 2 feet and have no joint limbs.) they create very sensitive and lyrical shadows, specially when they are animated by a peculiar jerky movement. The light source is produced by a bowl-shaped earthen lamp filled with castor-oil and three thick wicks made of cotton rags soaked in oil. This lamp is put on a stand of bamboo stick and an attached small wooden plank so adjusted that the lamp reaches to about 12 to 15 inches from the bottom of the screen. The distance between lamp and screen is at the most, 12 inches. The puppeteers sit on the ground and press different puppets into service in between the lamp and the screen. The leader of the group stands on the other side of the screen in full view of the audience. He holds in his hands a *khanjani*, a type of small tambourine cymbal and plays on it while singing. A vocalist often assists him from behind the screen. He and the manipulators behind the screen provide all the prose and impromptu dialogues for the puppets. The group usually consists of 4 members. The prose dialogues are delivered in recitative manner. The music is simple, but the words and vocal accompaniment are very much influenced by Odissi music. The theme is drawn exclusively from the Rama legend.

The shadow plays of Kerala locally known as *Tholpavakathu* are traditionally performed once a year during the annual temple festival. At other times they are performed as votive offerings commissioned by devotees. Like *Ravanchhaya* it also presents only the Rama legend and closely follows the Tamil *Kamba Ramayana*. The Kerala leather puppets have one joint hand which is manipulated particularly when the characters are engaged in conversation. In the Kerala shadow theatre a number of small earthen oil lamps provide several simultaneous light sources. With bamboo poles and the green bark of a banana plant a special stand is erected at a distance of about 12 inches from the screen running through the entire horizontal length reaching almost to the vertical centre. On this stand the oil lamps are put in a row spaced at about 6 to 9 inches from one another. The puppeteers stand behind the row of lamps and insert the puppets in between the lamp and the screen. The puppeteers themselves sing and deliver the prose dialogues. The musical accompanists also sit behind the screen. The group usually consists of 7 to 9 members. A long preliminary ritual precedes the show and the verbal aspect of the performance is highly operatic. Even the prose dialogues are delivered in a stylised manner. The music draws heavily upon the folk music of the region and carries traces of Karnataka classical influence.

Locally known as *Tholubomalatta*, the Andhra shadow play has the richest and the strongest tradition. The brightly coloured Andhra shadow-puppets are the largest of Indian puppets and are more versatile having joint shoulders, elbows, knees and sometime also waist, neck and ankles. The puppet-making craft follows an indigenous process in which the tanned leather is at first treated to a sort of translucency. Then the different parts of the puppet figure are cut out and are coloured with vegetable dyes according to traditional colour schemes. Finally, they are joined and a slim bamboo stick is tied to the puppet figure to keep it straight. For the light source, two iron brackets are hung from the ceiling of the puppet stage so that they reach the vertical point of the screen on both the sides. On these iron brackets either oil-soaked torches are lit or two huge lamps are lit. To facilitate manipulation the screen is slightly tilted towards the audience. The puppeteers then sing and deliver the prose dialogues while manipulating the puppets. In *Tholu-bomalatta*, the music is dominantly influenced by the classical music of the region and the theme for the puppet plays are drawn from Ramayana, Mahabharata and other Puranas.

The Karnataka shadow theatre, locally known as *Togalu Gombey-atta* is similar to that of Andhra in many respects. The puppets are equally colourful though a little smaller in size and in some cases a small scene is depicted by representing two or more characters in a single puppet. These highly decorative group figures are brought on to the screen like "freeze shots" to punctuate and intensify the dramatic effect. Themes for the Karnataka shadow plays are drawn from Ramayana, Mahabharata and other Puranic literatures as with the Andhra repertoire, with which it is related.

These inanimate figures manipulated by men once presented an extremely popular entertainment on village greens and street corners, fairs and festivals, in rustic barns and temple precincts. Their long history of unpretentious drama and simple mystery stretch right back to the dawn of our civilisation.

INDEX